# Brain Renovation
*Rebuild your brain from the ground up*

By

Benjamin Kramer
© Copyright 2014 Benjamin Kramer
4th Edition

# Table of Contents

## Introduction

Up until now, my publishing philosophy has been to slice my areas of expertise into small 'bite size' chunks and release them as short guides. My thinking was that someone who was interesting in increasing their levels of serotonin would not be particularly interested in a whole section on fixing their sleep, or vice versa.

However, recently, several people have suggested to me that the small guides I have published would all fit well into a broader book on brain health. You are now reading the result of these suggestions.

If you break down all the seemingly disparate topics which make up the broader subject of 'brain health', they will usually fall into the following catch-all categories -

- *fix your sleep*
- *eliminate stress*
- *consume 'brain building' nutrients*
- *eliminate 'brain toxic' foods and drugs*
- *use brain-specific supplements*
- *engage in 'brain healthy' behaviours*
- *engage in 'brain healthy' thought processes*

Taken as a whole, the purpose of this book is to help you rebuild a broken down brain or to ensure that you keep your brain from 'braking down' in the future by doing all the right things and avoiding a brain-toxic lifestyle.

The challenge in this book has been to slice and dice my original content to maintain clarity and to integrate brand new content not previously covered in the other guides I have written. The other challenge has been to cover a topic (such as meditation) which is applicable to more than one section. To use 'meditation' as an example, meditation is central to topics such as – increased serotonin, improved sleep, reduced stress and neural plasticity. So my challenge has been to cover certain topics multiple times in the book without repeating myself and boring the reader to death, which would be counter-productive to what I am trying to achieve! Hopefully I have met this challenge.

Good luck and a healthy brain to all!

*Benjamin Kramer*
*May 2014*

# Chapter 1 - Fix your sleep

Change Your Relationship with Sleep

This is by far the single most important aspect of fixing your sleep patterns and needs addressing before anything else.

Firstly, as an experiment, ask yourself the following question -

If I enjoyed being tired, would insomnia or poor quality sleep be an issue?

The answer, of course, is no.

Insomnia almost always follows the same pattern -

Difficulty falling asleep=>worried about being tired or functioning well the next day=>worry increases physiological response, making it more difficult to fall asleep=> and so on.

So before you proceed, you need to accept the fact that -

a)      Some nights you won't sleep well and you will feel a little under par the next day

b)      Your particular genetic, behavioural and psychological make-up means that you may find it difficult to fall asleep.  Just like someone with diabetes needs to accept this, so do you.  Fortunately, unlike Type 1 diabetes, there *is* something you can do to fix it.

This acceptance is a key first step because the more you struggle against your situation, the more you will suffer each night you struggle to get to sleep or sleep poorly.

Then you need to address the issue of how 'bad' you feel the next day after a poor night's sleep.  You need to 'stress test' this by asking yourself some key questions -

*If I sleep badly, exactly how 'bad' will I feel?  Describe the feeling.  How is it 'objectively' bad?  (i.e. - not just 'bad' because you don't want to feel that way)*

*What is the worst that could happen if I sleep poorly or don't get enough sleep?  Is it really so bad?*

The 8 Hour Myth

Probably the most dangerous piece of misinformation that is floated around is regarding the myth that we all need to get at least 8 hours sleep a night.  Not only is this biologically inaccurate, it is very dangerous information in the hands of the poor sleeper.  Insomniacs will, without fail, start to make calculations in their head based on what time it currently is and what time they have to wake up in the morning.  As this starts to hit the magical *'8 hour'* mark, physiological arousal increases, making it harder to sleep. The reason that this *"8 hour"* number is broadcast by health professionals is that as a general population, we are not allocating sufficient time for sleeping; choosing instead to work or party harder and *'sleep when I'm dead'*. The motivations for putting this number out there are good, however the subtleties are lost in the way the public receives this information.

Firstly, there is no fixed amount of sleep (or *'magic number'*) that everyone needs. Some people need 9 hours, some people 4. Many famous and productive people throughout history such as Margaret Thatcher, Thomas Edison & Bill Clinton got by on between 4 and 6 hours. Never set yourself a target on how many hours you need to sleep - this will only cause stress and make it harder to sleep. If you are sleep deprived for 1 night, your body has ingenious ways of making up the difference the following night. For example, it will prioritise slow-wave (deep) sleep in the night following sleep deprivation as this is the most important in terms of refreshing your body and brain. So even if you don't get *'8 hours'* the following night, it is likely that your sleep quality will be good.

There is something you can do as an experiment which you will find quite eye-opening. Choose a night where you do not have anything particularly taxing the next day which could make you stressed that night. Then, for that night, you need to make 'sleep *restriction*' your goal instead of trying to *maximise* your hours in bed. Remember, sleep restriction one night usually leads to good quality sleep the following night.

You will then discover several life-changing realisations -

Firstly, for the majority of people, the reason you feel bad after a night of insomnia is not the lack of *'hours'* in bed, but the worry and anxiety you experience before going to sleep. If you have a night where you deliberately only sleep 5 or 6 hours, you will find you actually don't feel so bad the next day. Think back to a time where you were having a lot of fun and only had a few hours of sleep - yet did not feel so bad the day after. For me, I think of those overnight flights overseas where you get 4 hours sleep or so. However, when you land at your destination, the excitement and enjoyment of a new country means you don't find the lack of sleep too troubling. My point is that a lack of sleep is not *fundamentally* bad - it is only the negative meanings you attach to it which make it so unpleasant.

The other realisation you will have is that when you try to restrict sleep, often you end up falling asleep more quickly. Sleep is strange like that - it seems to do the opposite to what you want. Try getting into bed and doing your best to fall asleep immediately and see what happens (*hint – it won't go well*). Your goal is to eventually reach a level of acceptance in your mind where you don't care how many hours sleep you get. Often the only difference between a good sleeper and a poor sleeper is that the poor sleeper has accumulated bad thought habits surrounding sleep. I used to be a poor sleeper and I was always amazed when someone said *"I only got 4 hours sleep last night"* and when you asked how they felt, they would say *"I'm ok, just a little tired"*. You realise that if it was you, it would be a 'disaster' and you 'wouldn't be able to function'. Your thoughts have become distorted and need correcting.

Sleep scientists refer to an approximately 6 hour portion of your nightly sleep as *'core sleep'*. Over a long period of time it is important you get at least your 'core sleep'. The hour or two over and above this helps for you to feel *'100%'* and thrive, however does not cause you any health related issues if you don't get it every night. Don't create scare stories in your mind that you will get cancer or go crazy if you don't get 8 hours sleep a night. Remember, a recent meta-analysis of various sleep research (a meta-analysis is when you pool different studies together to create a 'mega study' which should be more statistically accurate), showed that more than 9 hours sleep a night is associated with dying earlier than getting less than 8 hours sleep. Of course, this may mean that people sleeping more than 9 hours are doing so because their bodies are fighting a major illness, which leads to them dying earlier. However what is clear is that sleeping 9 or more hours a night does not make you healthier. *More is not always better.* Interestingly, for depressed people, restricting sleep can actually lead to a temporary improvement in mood. One of the reasons suggested is that major depression is associated with a large increase in REM sleep at the expense of slow wave sleep. Too much REM sleep can make you feel terrible as REM sleep is a similar state to being awake – it is not a period of sleep which contributes to your sense of feeling 'refreshed'. When you have an afternoon nap, unless you are seriously sleep deprived, your sleep will consist mainly of light sleep and REM sleep if you sleep longer than 20 mins. Remember how bad you felt after awakening from a long afternoon nap last time? That is how too much REM sleep feels. If your body has had enough slow wave sleep, your sleep mainly consists of light sleep and REM sleep and paradoxically, you feel more tired than if you had woken up an hour earlier.

## Have a hot bath before bed

I am not a fan of old wives tales or ineffectual solutions for insomnia. If you are a poor sleeper, a glass of milk or a cup of chamomile tea before bed is not going to do jack! However, one suggestion which is now backed by science is the recommendation to have a hot bath before bed.

This has been confirmed in a scientific study to increase slow wave sleep and subjective perception of sleep quality. The reason why a hot bath works is quite interesting.

There is a complex relationship between core body temperature and sleep. One of the things that scientists know, however, is that sleep is associated with a drop in body temperature. It is now believed that by artificially increasing core temperature via a hot bath, the natural decrease in body temperature which occurs after a hot bath sends a signal to your brain that it is time to sleep.

I have found this a little impractical during the hot months however in winter it works fantastically and I enjoy a great quality sleep. If you live in a tropical or sub-tropical location which is hot year round, I don't believe this is an option for you unless you spend all day in ice-cold air conditioning.

## Negative ions

Another one which sounds a little 'crackpot' until you verify the science is the idea that negative ions improve sleep quality. Multiple studies have tested whether either positively or negatively ionised air impacts sleep quality and the results are conclusive.

For example, one of the greatest known natural sources of positive ions is the *Santa Ana Winds* which blow across California. It has been shown that there is a statistically significant increase in murders and suicides when the winds are blowing. So what is the opposite of the *Santa Ana Winds*? A sea breeze which comes straight off the ocean. Think back to any time where you have slept right on the water or near the beach. I am willing to bet you slept like a log. However, there are many things at work here - not just ions. If you are sleeping near the beach there is a strong chance you are on holiday or relaxing. The sea air will also have all kinds of positive connotations for your brain in terms of nice memories.

However, even controlling for these factors there appears to be strong evidence favouring negative ions for sleep quality. If you don't live next to the beach, the best way to achieve this is via an ionizer which you set up in your bedroom. These can be expensive so this is only for those with the spare cash or with an interest in addressing every single aspect of their sleep issues. This is a 1%, icing on the cake tip and won't fix your sleep issues on its own.

## Avoid heavy meals in the evening

One of the easiest ways to mess up your sleep is to have a big heavy meal in the evening or a large snack straight before bed time. The physiological and hormonal situation in your body when you are digesting food is completely different to when your body is preparing itself for sleep. There is a complex relationship between insulin, cortisol and adrenaline which means digestion is incompatible with sleep.

Further to the hormonal reasoning, there is another major reason why you should not eat a large meal before bed - going to bed with a full stomach (maybe some heartburn or indigestion to go with it) is uncomfortable and an uncomfortable sleeper is a poor sleeper. If you are in discomfort, it will negatively affect your sleep quality. Anyone with a chronic pain condition will tell you this. If you can't get comfortable and pain free, your sleep will suffer.

Make your major meal lunch if possible. If you can't avoid a large meal in the evening, try to avoid simple carbohydrates which activate your insulin and cortisol system via your HPA (hypothalamic pituitary adrenal) Axis. Avoid pasta, bread and simple sugars where possible.

## Alcohol

Put simply, alcohol is the major sleep destroyer for the average person.

Different drugs (both prescription and recreational) affect sleep in different ways. However, apart from serious illegal drugs such as amphetamines and cocaine, alcohol has a unique ability to ruin sleep. This is for several major reasons.

Firstly, alcohol consumption in the evening causes you to spend more of your sleep time in light sleep, at the expense of slow wave and REM sleep. This is the main reason you wake up feeling sub-par after a night of even moderate drinking. As a side note, many chronic drinkers would read this comment and think "I sleep fine after drinking alcohol". However the fact is that if you drink alcohol every night, you would have forgotten what it is like to enjoy a solid night's sleep without alcohol affecting your sleep quality. After a period of abstinence, borderline alcoholics will often realise how much better sleep is without alcohol in their system.

Another problem alcohol causes is that, if you consume it during the evening, its effects wear of in the middle of the night while you are asleep and your body overcompensates by activating your brain. This often leads to awakenings which are then difficult to return to sleep from. Even if you do manage to get back to sleep, due to your increased level of physiological arousal, your sleep quality will be poor. This can be exacerbated by the fact that alcohol causes increase urination, so you can also expect to be awoken by your full bladder on multiple occasions.

Most poor sleepers I talk to are willing to do anything except quit alcohol. If you must consume alcohol, keep the volume low and keep your consumption as early as possible. A glass or two of beer or wine around 5pm shouldn't cause problems for too many people.

As a supplementary note, if you are a) suffering from depression and b) sleeping poorly and c) consuming alcohol in the evening, you really don't stand a chance and need to quit the alcohol as soon as possible. Alcohol plays havoc with serotonin, a key neurotransmitter involved in both mood and sleep which is implicated in major depression.

## Crank up your body's natural melatonin production

When there is no bright light hitting your eyes, it is a signal to the pineal gland to begin releasing melatonin, the sleep inducing hormone. Melatonin is vital to not only good quality sleep, but also to synchronising your body clock (your *circadian rhythm*). It is central to signalling your body to drop body temperature in readiness for sleep, as previously mentioned in the section on hot baths.

You may have heard of melatonin as a supplement you can buy in health-food stores, as it has become extremely popular for alleviating the symptoms of jet lag due to its body-clock resynchronising effects.

If you are a poor sleeper, you would be extremely surprised at how important it is for your room to be completely dark. Most people would think that the light coming in your room from a street light or other source of illumination in your room while you sleep would not be a major issue, however it can often be. Your body uses the sensation of light hitting your eyelids to control your body clock and wake you up.

If, for whatever reason, you cannot keep your room dark, invest in a high quality eye mask. When I travel, I use the *Infinity* brand, but any brand will do as long as it is a good quality mask which blocks out almost all light.

As your brain uses a lack of ambient light to signal that it is time to wind down and get ready for sleep, it is also vital to avoid unnecessarily bright lights in the couple of hours before bed also. Some people say that the modern day phenomenon of sleep problems is linked to the unnatural level of light we experience in the evening before bed. It is believed that in ancient history, due to a lack of electricity, humans would sleep soon after sun down and awaken at dawn. Or perhaps they spent a little time in the evening, socialising by campfire or candlelight. One thing is for certain - they did not spend the hour before bed looking at a computer or television screen.

I strongly recommend you remove all bright sources of light after 8pm. Make sure the house only has lamps on for mood and try to turn the TV or computer off as early as possible. Consider spending the time before bed meditating or reading something by dim light (see upcoming sections).

Go to bed and wake up at the same time each day

As you read previously, melatonin controls your body clock to tell your brain when to sleep and when to wake up, however you also need to give it some help. It is vital that you go to bed and wake up at the same time each day. This will condition your brain and your circadian rhythm for quality sleep.

This is clear to see when you stay up later than normal and then wake up later than normal. Even though you may have had the same amount of sleep, you feel tired all day. This is because you are awake when your brain thinks you should be asleep and asleep when you should be awake. For example, in the early morning, your body starts to produce cortisol to prepare you to wake up. If you continue to sleep with elevated cortisol in your bloodstream, your quality of sleep will not be good. Cortisol is also produced in response to stress and is elevated in people with major depression or an anxiety disorder. This may partly explain the poor sleep quality experienced by these people.

People who suffer insomnia tend to do the same thing - if they are up late at night because they can't get to sleep, they will sleep later, in the misguided belief that this will enable them to 'make up' their lost hours. However this only makes the situation worse.

During the day, your brain builds up *'sleep pressure'* - meaning - that the longer you are awake, the greater the body's urge to sleep is. It does this primarily via the substance *adenosine* (coffee and other caffeinated beverages work by inhibiting the action of adenosine). If you stay away for 24 hours, when you eventually sleep, you would be asleep within moments and the quality of your sleep would be good. If you slept in past your usual waking time, by the time your usual sleeping time came around later that night, you wouldn't have been awake long enough to have built up much sleep pressure. This creates an endless cycle of poor sleeping.

The solution?  Even if you are up late, make sure you get up the same time as usual.  Yes you will be tired that day, but come bed time, you will enjoy a fantastic sleep as your body tries to make up for the previous night's deficit.

Same goes for when you go to bed.  If you have been sleeping poorly and feel the urge to go to bed earlier than usual to make up for lost time, don't do it.  You won't have enough sleep pressure and you run the risk of just lying in bed and starting the cycle all over.

While on the subject of sleep pressure, let me address the topic of 'naps'.  This is a controversial topic with a few different viewpoints.  Some sleep specialists thing afternoon naps are ok as long as you keep them under 20 minutes.  The reason for 20 minutes is that after this period you transition from light sleep into deeper stages (predominantly REM for afternoon naps) which will leave you feeling terrible and groggy when you wake up.  Also, if you have a long afternoon nap, you will not have enough sleep pressure later that evening when you go to bed.  These sleep specialists believe that this is the evolutionary function for that 2pm 'slump' people get where they suddenly feel like sleeping in the afternoon.

However other sleep specialists believe that naps are to be avoided at all costs as they compromise your circadian rhythm and reduce sleep pressure.

At the end of the day, see what works for you.  It will be extremely clear what works and what doesn't work.  In my case, particularly on a beach holiday, slowly falling asleep in the afternoon while reading or relaxing is one of the nicest feelings in the world.  However if I go past that magical 20 minute mark, I am a disaster for the rest of the day and don't sleep as well that night.

Exercise to improve your sleep

As mentioned in the section on hot baths, body temperature is integrally related to the quality of your sleep.  The ideal pattern for good sleep is a body temperature that rises in the late afternoon or early evening and then falls later in the evening before bed.

A natural way to stimulate this important rise in body temperature is to exercise vigorously.  Any type of exercise is fine, as long as it gets your heart rate up and your blood pumping

The other way that exercise is beneficial for sleep is via the effects on various neurotransmitters.  This area involves a little speculation and debate as to what it is about exercise that improves sleep.  One of the hypotheses is that it involves a release of calming neurotransmitters and hormones such as serotonin and endorphins which improve sleep.  Another idea is that intense exercise burns through adrenaline (the body's key stimulating neurotransmitter), leading to post-exercise relaxation.

Whatever the actual underlying reason, the fact remains that exercise is a key weapon in your fight against poor sleep.

One key point that needs addressing though is timing. Playing a game of soccer which finishes an hour before bed time will be counterproductive and lead to worse sleep, not better. The reason for this is that your body needs time for your core temperature to drop back down again. It is therefore recommended that you finish exercising at least six hours before bed time. Six hours appears to be the magic sweet spot in terms of exercise improving sleep. More on exercise soon...

## Naps

The topic of naps in sleep science is a controversial one. Some sleep scientists believe that naps are counterproductive, some believe they are beneficial. At the end of the day you should do whatever is best in terms of your overall sleep quality and daytime functioning.

Naps form a central part of the lives of people in certain countries. In particular, the afternoon 'siesta' has been made famous by the Spanish (and other Spanish speaking countries). Some sleep scientists believe that this is the 'natural' rhythm for humans as it matches that 'slump' many people experience after lunch where the idea of a nap becomes so enticing. They believe that by having a brief nap in the afternoon, you are sticking to your body's natural circadian rhythm.

For those who use naps successfully, the key is definitely duration and timing. Any daytime nap should be kept to twenty minutes maximum. This is for two main reasons. If you nap for longer than this, you risk having no sleep pressure later that evening, which will result in poor quality sleep. Secondly, if you nap for longer than twenty minutes you will go into the deeper stages of sleep. This means that when you finally wake up you will be groggy and tired for the rest of day.

In terms of timing, the key is to keep it to a brief nap early in the afternoon. Any later than this and you will definitely have a negative impact on your sleep quality later that evening.

The other key factor which should impact your decision whether to nap or not is whether you are actually sleep deprived or not. If you are uncomfortably sleepy due to a lack of sleep or poor sleep the night before, a quick nap could really perk you up for the rest of the day. If you are perfectly rested and not tired at all, perhaps a nap would not be in your best interests – particularly if you are trying to build up sleep pressure for later that night.

## Only use your bed for sleep and 'sweet lovin'

This is a common and useful tip. Your brain needs to associate your bed with sleep and, to a lesser extent, sex (or to a greater extent if you are really lucky). If you do all kinds of other activities in your bed such as emails, net surfing or planking, your brain will be confused about context. Make it so that when you lay down in bed, your subconscious knows exactly what you are there for. Subtle cues will then make you sleepy. This one is easy.

## Meditation

Learning to meditate is really a no-brainer as there are so many positive benefits for your mind and body. It increases levels of feel good neurotransmitters such as serotonin and reduces levels of stress hormones such as cortisol, which is often chronically elevated in people with long term sleep issues.

*Why is meditation so important for sleep?*

Firstly, one of the major determinants of the quality of your sleep is your level of physiological arousal prior to going to bed. If you go to bed immediately after watching a gripping horror movie or having a nasty argument with someone, the quality of your sleep will not be good. Contrast this to how you sleep when you are on holidays or not stressed at work.

Meditation is proven to be without equal in terms of reducing physiological arousal. Study after study shows it is more effective than other relaxation methods for reducing heart rate and galvanic skin response. So meditating prior to bed will not only improve the quality of your sleep but make it easier to fall asleep also.

Secondly, several studies have indicated that meditation can actually *replace* some of your sleep. Your brain wave pattern in deep meditation has a striking similarity with certain stages of actual sleep. I have spoken to many long term meditators who generally indicate that 20 minutes of deep meditation is worth at least 1 or 2 hours sleep. This is good to know if you are still stressing yourself over getting 8 hours sleep a night. If you are having difficulty sleeping, you can do some meditation in the knowledge that you are recharging your brain, even if you are not actually asleep. As I touched on previously, one of the reasons you feel so bad after a night of insomnia is the anxiety and stress it causes, impacting sleep quality. If you know you can just perch yourself up in bed, or find a nice comfortable chair and meditate for a while, this will dramatically reduce your stress levels. You can even reframe the whole situation when if you have trouble falling asleep - "*Ah, here is another opportunity to practice meditation*".

There are thousands of books and websites giving instructions on how to meditate so it is pointless in me giving a detailed explanation of the whole topic so I will concentrate on giving you the basics. However I encourage you to dig deeper into this topic as the benefits extend beyond just improved sleep.

For a quick and easy seated meditation technique, visit Appendix 1

An alternative to seated meditation is to meditate while still lying down. If you do this there is a strong chance it will send you off to sleep quickly. However one downside is you don't get a break from laying down. You may have read the advice that if you can't get to sleep you should get up out of bed and do something for a while before returning to bed when you are sleepy. Even just getting out of bed and getting a small drink or snack can often be enough so that when you get back into bed you fall straight asleep. To be honest, no one knows for sure why this is so, but it works. My theory is that after a while laying down in bed without getting to sleep, you become a little more uncomfortable than when you got in to bed. Think about that moment you get into bed after a long, tiring day. After a while the pleasant sensation fades. I think that be getting out of bed for a while you have a chance to reset this so that when you get back into bed you are once again comfortable and fall asleep soon after.

## Reading before bed

I am a big fan of reading before bed for a few reasons. Firstly, it is a great alternative to looking at a TV or computer screen before you sleep. Especially if you read by a nice dim, warmly lit (i.e. - not fluorescent) lamp.

Secondly, you can carefully choose non-arousing (physiological arousal, not sexual) reading materials. In my opinion, the best options are light fiction or religious/spiritual materials. For fiction, you need to avoid Thrillers, Horror or anything else exciting. You don't want 'exciting' before bed. For non-fiction, I like reading books on Zen Buddhism which never have anything particularly exciting; perfect for pre-bed reading! If you are not spiritually inclined, pick a subject which is not too intellectually taxing or psychologically stimulating.

## Supplements for better sleep

Supplements are not going to do all the work for you so don't expect to just take a pill each night and you are cured. In fact, sometimes I avoid even suggesting supplements because they can be disempowering for people with insomnia. What do I mean by this? If you take a tablet, subconsciously your brain knows it hasn't conquered insomnia and it is just a temporary fix. When you then stop taking a tablet and you have failed to address the causes of your insomnia, you will just return to sleeping poorly.

However if you are doing all the other important things, supplements can provide some nice assistance to getting a good night's sleep. However, remember, supplements are not sleeping pills - the effects are much more mild, so for cases of severe sleep issues, they will be ineffectual. Here are some I recommend to help mild sleep issues -

| | |
|---|---|
| *Valerian -* | The gold standard of herbal sleeping supplements |
| *Passionflower -* | Helps reduce anxiety and improve sleep |
| *5-htp -* | 5htp is an amino-acid precursor to serotonin so if serotonin issues are behind your sleep problems, this can help |
| *Withania Somnifera (Ashwaghanda) -* | A popular *ayurvedic* herb which has all kinds of benefits for your brain, not just improved sleep. Often lumped in the dubious 'adaptogen' category however withania has documented benefits. |

Medications for difficult cases

In general, medications should be viewed as either a temporary solution or a long term solution in rare cases where there is no improvement and quality of life is being impacted. Many of them give a poor quality of sleep and can have side-effects which may be intolerable. However you need to be pragmatic. If you and your doctor are comfortable that you have exhausted all non-pharmaceutical options to no avail, medication can be a life saver for some.

The most common type of sleeping pill is one in the benzodiazepine class. These are the ones that end in "am". Such as -

- *Alprazolam (Xanax)* - very powerful, used more for anxiety than sleep disorders but very effective
- Diazepam (Valium) - an effective sleeping pill
- *Temazepam (Restoril)* - another common sleeping pill

There are several problems with this class of drug. Firstly, the quality of sleep they give is terrible. They rob you of valuable REM and slow wave sleep, your two most important stages. They consequently can leave you feeling worse the next day than if you hadn't slept at all. Strangely though, for the chronically anxious, this class of medication can leave some people feeling fantastic the day after, as they are powerful anxiety killers.

Secondly, they can abused or be habit forming for some people. Personally I think the risk of psychological addiction for the general population is low. Unless you are anxious or trying to dull some strong psychological pain in your life, these drugs have limited recreational potential or risk of abuse in my opinion.

Thirdly, if you use them for more than a few days or weeks, or escalate the dose, you *will* become physically addicted to them. This means that you will have to slowly reduce (or 'taper') your dose to avoid health issues. Believe it or not, stopping an addiction to this class of drugs is significantly more dangerous than stopping Heroin as there is risk or seizure or death. That alone should form enough of a warning to avoid using these for more than a few days or in emergencies. Further to this, long term use of Benzodiazepines is associated with a decline in cognitive function; something you probably want to avoid if possible.

However in the last couple of decades, pharmaceutical companies have made several refinements to benzodiazepines to create more specific drugs including *Zolpidem (Ambien)* and *Eszopiclone (Lunesta)*. These drugs specifically work on the exact receptor subtypes (of the brain's GABA receptors primarily) so that they put you to sleep but without the other effects of Benzodiazepines. These medications are believed to be safer for long term use, however do not 'cure' your sleep problems. This class of drugs is mainly for people who have problems initially falling asleep. They do not improve poor quality sleep for most people. Indeed, due to their short half-life (i.e. - the effectiveness wears off after a few hours), many people complain that they suddenly wake up in the middle of the night and cannot get back to sleep. Each of these drugs vary in their half-life so in general, choose a longer half-life if you wake up in the middle of the night and a shorter half-life if you wake up the next morning groggy (as you are still under the effects of the drug).

## Anti-histamine Class

Most 'over the counter' (OTC) sleep aids consist of an anti-histamine of some description. The most popular are - *promethazine, diphenhydramine* and *doxylamine.* I have found that people either love them or hate them for sleep. Many people don't like them as they still feel groggy the next day. The benefits over benzodiazepines is that anti-histamines in general, actually improve your sleep architecture. For example, a rarely used anti-histamine called *cyproheptadine* actually increases slow wave sleep.

Apart from improved sleep quality, the other main benefit of anti-histamines is a lack of addictive qualities and proven long term safety. Anti-histamines are almost unique in their lack of adverse health impact among most medicines. Furthermore, I have never heard any incidence of 'addiction' to anti-histamines.

However, using these long term still doesn't fix your sleep issues. You are still taking a tablet to reduce 'symptoms' rather than addressing any underlying cause.

## Sedating antidepressants

These can be particularly helpful if your insomnia is caused by anxiety or depression as they can address both.

In my experience, the best of this class is mirtazapine (Remeron) as it has the best safety profile. If you look at how mirtazapine works in your brain, it is really just an anti-histamine plus weak antidepressant. However, in general it is safe to take long term however, as with everything else, try to avoid staying on it indefinitely. For some people it can lead to significant weight gain (both via water retention and increased appetite).

The other option in this class is the old style tricyclics (TCAs) such as amitriptyline or imipramine. Unless you are anxious, depressed or in pain (they also decrease certain types of pain) I would stay away from these. The side effect profile is horrendous with a long list of nasty side effects such as weight gain, dry mouth, fatigue and cardio-toxicity (they are bad for your heart). Last but not least, if you take too many at once you can overdose and die.

Another option to investigate in this class is *trazodone (Desyrel)*, however this medication is only available in certain markets. It works in a similar way to Mirtazapine and many people find it helpful for sleep problems.

## Anticonvulsants

The drugs *gabapentin (Neurontin)* and *pregabalin (Lyrica)* are an interesting and rarely used option for improving sleep as they specifically improve slow wave sleep. They are mainly used for Fibromyalgia however could also be considered as an option for poor sleep quality. As with mirtazapine, main side effect is weight gain however some people also report some cognitive decline on high doses or with long-term treatment.

## Fix any underlying issues affecting your sleep

To take a step backwards, in many cases sleep problems are a symptom of broader issues in your life. The most common of these are relationship and work problems. To fix your sleep you need to resolve these issues. The brain does not like going to sleep with major issues unresolved and this can gradually lead to chronically poor sleep if the issue does not get addressed. If you are in a toxic relationship, get out. If you are in a good relationship with some specific issue causing friction, resolve it. If you hate your job and you can afford to quit, quit. If you can't afford to quit, get pro-active about fixing the situation at work or finding a better job.

Scientists have found one of the surest triggers of depression and anxiety is helplessness. If you put a mouse in a situation where it is electrocuted and has no way to control the shocks, it will soon display the symptoms of anxiety and depression. If you feel helpless about some aspect of your life, take control. The simple act of taking control will completely change both your mind-set and physiological status, leading eventually to improved sleep. But it will take time for your brain to learn new, healthy sleep habits.

## Chapter 2 – Rebuild your brain using the power of neuroplasticity

*What is Brain (or Neuro) Plasticity?*

Put simply, until only recently, scientists believed that after childhood, the brain was fixed and unchangeable. However that belief has now been turned on its head thanks to recent advances in neural imaging such as fMRI (Functional Magnetic Resonance Imaging).

FMRI scans have clearly demonstrated that the adult brain has the clear ability to re-organize itself based on the experiences of the person. The classic example given is – if you scan the brain of a musician, the part of their brain responsible for controlling the instrument (such as a cello) is much larger and more active than a non-musician.

Why is this so important? You can use this concept for many aspects of your life such as –

- Cure depression and anxiety (or at least alleviate its severity)

- Improve your focus & attention

- Improve your sleep quality

- Improve your general health

- Increase your intelligence

This is NOT a quick-fix solution to your troubles – to utilize neuro plasticity takes time and effort. You must break old habits – both mental and behavioural.

So we know that this requires repetitive activity with conscious effort, so what are the best ways to utilize neuro plasticity to make meaningful changes to your brain?

- Cognitive behavioural therapy (CBT)

- Meditation & Buddhist psychology

- Exercise

- Yoga

These are the major headline topics however I will also cover promising emerging concepts as the evidence becomes clearer. I will also try to keep this book as simple and jargon-free as possible. One of the things I aim to achieve with this book is to condense the information I get from various sources into easy to understand lay terms. So often I have found the most fascinating piece of information buried under pages and pages of barely understandable 'research talk'.

Before we proceed I need to make an extremely important point which is applicable to almost everything in this book – the key to any activity I mention is *attention*. In the majority of cases, neuroplasticity requires focussed, directed attention to be effective. Naturally, this goes without saying in the case of meditation. If you are not focussed while meditating, you are not meditating! However, this is also the case for most other things I mention. Attention is the magnifying glass which concentrates everything into a laser beam. Don't do anything in this book while you are distracted as you will need to apply 100% of your attention to each of the activities to extract full value.

## Change Your Thinking

Changing your thinking is, I believe, the single most important factor in changing the way your brain is wired. However it is also the aspect which takes the most effort and the longest time. Behaviours are relatively easy to change with a little effort. Faulty thought habits are notoriously difficult to erase and replace.

*Cognitive Behavioural Therapy (CBT)* is now the gold-standard psychotherapy for this very reason as it is without equal in terms of a structured system for changing faulty thinking. CBT is best done with the guidance of a qualified therapist, not via a book. However I will touch on some of the basic principles which you can apply to your own situation.

Disorders such as anxiety and depression are characterised by what is known as 'maladaptive' thought processes which do not stand up to logical assessment. Here are some classic examples –

- Your boss gets angry with you for something and you then assume you are going to be fired

- You get a panic attack when you are around a big crowd of people – even though you know there is nothing that will harm you

- You have a fear of flying – despite a logical understanding of the probability that you will crash

The majority of all maladaptive thought issues centre on the concept of 'catastrophizing'. This essentially involves getting a small piece of information and then extrapolating it to the worse possible outcome. Some perfect examples –

- You get a headache and immediately think that it is a brain tumour

- You won't talk in public because you think that you will have a panic attack and everyone will laugh at you

At the heart of depression and anxiety usually lie at least some elements of catastrophizing. The best way to tackle this is with the power of logic, particularly by employing elements of S*ocratic questioning*. Here are some questions to ask yourself about a particular scenario or situation –

*What is the likelihood of it occurring?*

*What is the highest probability outcome?*

*If the feared event transpires, what is the absolute worst that can happen?*

*What evidence do you have to support your view?*

After practicing this for a while, you should soon have the two following realisations –

*The things you fear rarely eventuate*

*If they do eventuate, it is rarely as bad as you thought it would be*


One of the hallmarks of poor mental health is a kind of permanent *negative filter* on everything you perceive. Things that gave you pleasure in the past are no longer enjoyable. You dread safe and neutral events. You misinterpret neutral, offhand remarks made by others. One of the best ways to start removing this negative filter is to first realise that the majority of events are neither good nor bad – there is only your interpretation of the events. For example, pretend that your spouse announces that they want a divorce. Is this good or bad? What if you were in love with another person and had been trying to work up the courage to break up with your spouse?

It's all about context. That is why the *hippocampus* is so strongly involved in anxiety and depression, as it is responsible for attributing context to events. The *hippocampi* of depressed people often demonstrate some degree of atrophy, showing less activity than a non-depressed person. Fortunately the *hippocampus* is one of the most plastic parts of your brain, responding well to a positive change in thinking and behaviour. Interestingly, SSRI medication has also been shown to positively change the *hippocampus*, perhaps indicating one of the reasons for therapeutic effectiveness.

Buddhism tells us that we suffer due to attachment and ignorance. We are *attached* to certain events and when they do not occur, we suffer. Furthermore, we become attached to things due to our ignorance of the true reality. The following old Chinese story is a great example of this –

*One day a farmer's only horse runs away.*

*"How terrible!" says the neighbour*

*"Good, bad, who knows?" says the farmer*

*The next day the horse returns with several new horses*

*"How wonderful!" says the neighbour*

*"Good, bad, who knows?" says the farmer*

*The next day, while trying to break in the new horses, the farmer's only son breaks his leg*

*"How terrible!" says the neighbour*

*"Good, bad, who knows?" says the farmer*

*The next day, the army visits the farm to conscript young men for war; however the farmer's son is saved due to his broken leg*

*"How wonderful!" says the neighbour*

*"Good, bad, who knows?" says the farmer*

You need to consider whether you may have slowly developed the habit of attributing negative meaning to events which may not be so. How many people have said that a particular event which they thought was devastating at the time, eventually proved to be a blessing? So many people have lost their jobs, only to discover their true calling. Or have been divorced from their spouse, only to meet the love of their life?

## Meditation and mindfulness
Meditation has innumerable benefits, such as –

- reduced stress

- improved sleep

- reduced anxiety

- improved physical health – such as lower blood pressure

From a neurological perspective, meditation is one of the best activities you can engage in to foster neural plasticity.

However I should note that meditation is not recommended for the acute stage of a depressive or anxious disorder. If you are not an experienced meditator it can actually make you more agitated if you are not used to simply sitting and being with your thoughts. Exercise is a far better option for these stages as it gives the opposite – sweet distraction!

Meditation is no quick fix – in fact the mindset behind meditation is almost the exact opposite from taking a pill – there is no easy 'pop a pill' option – you have to work at it – but the rewards are immense. *Ram Dass*, the Harvard professor who, along with *Timothy Leary*, introduced LSD to America in the 1960s, likened drug experiences to being able to briefly visit heaven in an artificial sense. However, after realising the emptiness of the drug experience compared to meditation and spiritual practices, he said that meditation was a way to stay in heaven, not just visit briefly. Similarly, meditation can be a way to completely obviate the need for medication in the long run – but it <u>will</u> take time. Patience must be cultivated.

Again, for a quick and easy seated meditation technique, visit <u>Appendix 1</u>

One of the greatest benefits of meditation in this context is that it slowly builds up a separation between 'me' and 'my thoughts'. You gradually develop a kind of $3^{rd}$ person perspective with your thoughts which can take the emotional sting out of them. This means that meditation is a great companion to CBT as it gives you the techniques to better monitor faulty thought processes and to not get caught up in your thoughts so much.

The practice of mindfulness brings an additional dimension to your meditative practice. Mindfulness has been popularised by identities such as *Dr Jon Kabat Zinn* and Zen monk *Thich Nhat Hanh*. I strongly encourage you to seek out their work (some selected books will be listed in the Recommended Reading section).

Mindfulness essentially involves bringing a kind of *'non-judgemental'* awareness to your physical and mental states. It acknowledges that there are all kinds of filters which we put on experience which just add to suffering. The best example is pain. Pain is simply a sensation in the body which is there to get your attention. As much as we dislike pain, the alternative can be much worse. There are a group of people with a genetic mutation which causes them to feel no pain. These people end up losing limbs and dying early as they do not have the body's natural warning system – pain.

Due to its importance for our survival, pain has been given a very strong connection to our emotional centres such as the *limbic system*. One of the valuable applications of mindfulness is in the area of pain relief. Mindfulness can involve learning to look at pain dispassionately – as just a sensation. Put another way, when we feel pain, there is the actual physical sensation and then there is the mental suffering which then occurs. This mental suffering is not only unpleasant, but has been shown to intensify the sensation of pain. For many conditions you cannot eliminate pain, however if you can tone down your emotional reaction to it, the physical sensation of pain usually also reduces in intensity.

Change your behaviour
Each of the topics in this section on neural plasticity can be considered like legs on a table – neglect one of them and you are going to struggle to keep the table standing.

Behaviour is no different. You can do everything outlined in this book perfectly except fix your behaviour and it will be a waste of time.

*"Behaviourism"* dominated the field of psychology for so long for the simple fact that addressing your behaviour is a key aspect of healing your brain. Where pure *'Behaviourism'* fell down was how it neglected the *"cognitive"* side, hence the advent of CBT. However that does not mean that the behavioural aspect is not important – it is central to a healthy brain and to the ability to rebuild a broken brain.

## Get social

Humans are designed to socialise – we are not *'lone wolves'*. It has even been suggested by some evolutionary biologists that humans developed our *pre-frontal cortex (PFC)* to enable us to navigate complex social networks. When you see someone who struggles in life due to a lack of PFC control over their limbic system, you can easily understand this hypothesis.

This point I can't stress strongly enough – one of the single greatest thing you can do to maintain a healthy brain and to rebuild a broken one is to force yourself to socialise. This may seem counterintuitive as one of the hallmarks of depression is a tendency to avoid people and stay at home. It may not be easy, but you have to force yourself to get out – go to a party, hang out with friends, play sport – whatever gets you out of the house and interacting with other people.

Socialising with others stimulates the release of all kinds of 'feel-good' hormones such as Serotonin and Oxytocin. Laughing with friends has also been shown to stimulate the production of Endorphins. On top of the neurochemistry, interacting with others occupies your mind in a positive way, preventing you from sitting around and ruminating about your troubles.

## Exposure & Avoidance

There is an old saying which is incredibly salient – "*A fear avoided is a fear doubled*". For people suffering from anxiety, *avoidance behaviours* are one of the most insidious aspects of their illness, as each time the sufferer avoids a situation, they are reinforcing the fear. If you have a mild fear of flying and you start avoiding flying anywhere, pretty soon you will have a fully blown phobia.

The reason is that when you avoid something, it is sending a signal to your primitive fear centres of your brain that this is something dangerous and your brain needs to look out for it in future. This is helpful when it relates to a snake or tiger, but less so if it involves a phobia about flying.

The early Behaviourists recognised this and utilised exposure therapy to extinguish these phobias. If you have a fear of spiders, you would start by looking at pictures of spiders in a book, gradually work up to seeing them in real life and maybe get to the point where you will touch one (a harmless one of course). Each exposure slowly rebuilds your brain to eradicate the illogical phobia.

So the key messages are –

- Never avoid situations due to illogical fear
- Create controlled exposure scenarios with whatever you are fearful of

## Nutrition and supplements to rebuild your brain
*Feed Your Brain Quality Fuel*

Whilst I don't believe it is quite as crucial as some other aspects for rebuilding your brain, the right nutrition is also an important piece of the puzzle. I am going to start by being incredibly boring – the single most important thing you can do in this area is to eat a balanced diet with plenty of fruit, vegetables and animal protein.

You will notice that I did not mention grains or legumes. This is a slightly controversial point however the weight of research has been recently turning against grains and legumes. They are simply not that great for your body, 'wholegrain' or not. They contain a whole raft of problematic substances such as *protease inhibitors*, *phytic acid* and other *anti-nutritional factors*. These prevent the absorption of vital minerals and protein.

Herein lies the problem of vegetarianism and veganism. The ethics of following this lifestyle are beyond reproach. To take a stand against the harming of animals is admirable. I, on the other hand, am significantly more cowardly. I eat meat, yet I can't bear to think about an animal getting killed to feed me. Once, as part of a job I had, I was forced to visit an abattoir once and found it extremely distressful and couldn't watch the part where the cow was slaughtered. Some people say that if you eat meat, you should be forced to kill it yourself or at least witness it and this argument has theoretical (if not practical) merit.

However, the purpose of this book is to get you healthy again and for that, if you don't eat any meat, you are going to be at a significant disadvantage. Firstly, vegetable protein (such as soy) is just not very well absorbed by the human body compared to animal protein. Blame those protease inhibitors and other anti-nutritional factors. Secondly, a vegetarian or vegan diet which replaces animal protein with grain and legumes is going to have a poor omega 3 to omega 6 ratio. This sets you up for inflammation or a worsening of any existing inflammation. I will talk more about these essential fatty acids soon. Thirdly, you will not be getting a diverse and complete range of essential amino-acids.

All the amino-acids are vital in one way or another however the two key amino-acids involved in the biogenesis of depression and anxiety are tryptophan and tyrosine.

Why is tryptophan so important? It is the key building block of serotonin, so if you do not consume enough of it, you are not giving your brain the best chance possible. Eggs, cheese and various meats are high in tryptophan. Soybeans also contain tryptophan however those pesky protease inhibitors make these a questionable source of tryptophan.

Tyrosine is used for the manufacturer of dopamine and noradrenaline, two other key neurotransmitters. Again, whilst you can get some tyrosine from certain nuts and fruit, animal protein is the richest source.

Vegetarian diets are also famous for requiring B12 injections due to the lack of red meat being consumed. B12 is vital for the normal functioning of many parts of the body but particularly the brain. If you are trying to get your brain healthy, a B12 deficient diet simply is not an option.

So, if you are a vegetarian and have read above yet would still like to persist with that particular lifestyle, it is completely your choice. However, remember that you made that choice knowing the potential consequences. To be clear, I am not saying that no-one can thrive on a vegetarian diet. For example, Buddhist monks are known to subsist on a primarily vegetarian diet and rarely have any issues (a notable exception being the Dalai Lama!). However they are in a non-stressed state with different nutritional requirements. Likewise, many vegetarians get by just fine and there are even some high-level athletes who are vegetarian. Remember, you are trying to fix your brain and animal protein and omega 3 fatty acids are a key factor in that.

## Essential Fatty Acids

If I was to be forced to pick the single most important 'nutrient' for the brain it would be omega 3 fatty acids. The brain is comprised largely of omega 3 and requires sufficient quantities of it in your diet to repair and rebuild the brain. Omega 3 is mainly comprised of DHA and EPA. It is DHA which is most important for the brain – in fact, DHA has been demonstrated to stimulate neurogenesis, similar to the effects of BDNF.

As you would probably know, the major source of omega 3 in the diet is from seafood and in particular, fatty fish like salmon. However, most people think that simply having a diet with sufficient omega 3 is enough, which isn't the case. The most important aspect is your overall ratio of omega 3 to omega 6 consumption. Put simply, omega 3 is anti-inflammatory and omega 6 is pro-inflammatory. When the ratio gets out of whack, inflammation results. The average western diet has an omega 6 to omega 3 ratio of around 20:1. It is believed that humans evolved on a diet with a ratio of closer to 1:1. What is driving this change? Yes, our old friends - grains and legumes. Not only are we replacing foods high in omega 3 with grains such as wheat, we are also cooking our food in vegetable oil (such as canola and soybean oil) high in omega 6. This is further exacerbated by the red meat and chicken we now eat. Historically, cows grazed on grasses rich in omega 3 ("grass fed"), however they are now fed largely on grains and legumes such as corn, soybean meal and feed wheat, thus increasing the omega 6 content of the meat.

If you want a healthy brain and you love red meat, you need to seek out grass-fed beef. However, at the end of the day, seafood still remains the obvious, low risk choice. Just avoid the fish at the top of the food chain like shark, tuna & swordfish as they can contain high levels of mercury – perhaps the most toxic substance known for the brain. You can't go wrong with common choices like salmon or sardines.

So, in the interest of simplicity, let me give the following dietary guidelines for a healthy brain -

– Eat unlimited quantities of vegetables – particularly leafy greens which are high in folate, a key co-factor in the production of serotonin

– Eat unlimited quantities of low-fructose fruits such as berries. Many of today's fruits have been bred for sweetness (*read – high fructose*). Don't think you can gorge on unlimited quantities of apples or bananas. A fruit-heavy diet contains huge amounts of fructose which taxes your adrenal system – the opposite of what you want to be doing

– Following on from this, limit sugar consumption for the same reason. Also, avoid anything containing flour (wheat or corn) which is essentially the same as eating sugar.

– Don't try to limit the consumption of good fats. Avoid omega 6 and trans-fats. Here is where I am going to get controversial – don't worry about consuming saturated fat. Saturated fat is vital for all kinds of biological processes and has gotten an undeserved bad rap. It drives me crazy whenever I see the expression "*artery clogging fat*" as this is a gross simplification. When people say this, the first thing I say is "When you diet, your body is liberating saturated fat from your fat deposits to burn for fuel and we don't call this '*artery clogging*' do we?" If you need further proof, look at traditional communities who consume huge amounts of saturated fat such as the Inuit and the *Maasai*. They have next to no incidence of heart disease, except where they have been introduced to western food such as wheat flour and sugar.

– Eat varied sources of animal protein - mainly seafood

– Avoid – grains and legumes.

– For dairy, it depends on the person. The ability to tolerate lactose (the main sugar in dairy) was a genetic mutation which occurred in northern Europeans in reasonably recent history. If your genetics or state of health allows you to consume dairy, go for it. If not, stay away from it. Don't believe the advertising of the milk industry – milk doesn't contain anything you can't get elsewhere (such as calcium)

– If you are recovering from mental illness or a period of high stress, or if you have a general sensitivity, avoid alcohol completely. For a depressed alcohol lover, this is the hardest advice to follow. Many people would subconsciously rather stay depressed than give up alcohol. However the fact remains that alcohol is terrible for the brain. It temporarily raises serotonin (making you feel good), before levels crash later (leaving you feel terrible). It completely ruins your sleep architecture, keeping you in light sleep. Not the best combination for someone trying to heal their brain.

– Eggs are a miracle food. They do NOT 'increase your cholesterol, leading to increased heart disease risk'.  This is a simplistic and out dated idea which has been disproven (that consuming cholesterol increases your serum cholesterol – particularly LDL)

# Chapter 3 - Improve your mood via Increased Serotonin

Now I know what you many of my readers may think when they read a whole sections dedicated to serotonin – *what about noradrenaline (norepinephrine) and dopamine?* Well, firstly, I think many of the suggestions in this section are applicable to all the monoamines (and potentially the stress hormones as well) so if you follow the advice in this section, you should see optimized levels of all. Secondly, out of all the monoamines, I believe serotonin to be the most likely to suffer from sub-optimal levels, hence the requirement for greater focus on this important neurotransmitter.

Since the advent of *Prozac* (and subsequent medicines in the SSRI class), serotonin really has been the hottest neurotransmitter on the block!

Before *Prozac*, the focus of most drugs was on increasing levels of the three main neurotransmitters implicated in mental illness - noradrenaline (or norepinephrine in certain countries), dopamine and serotonin.

The previous types of antidepressants - *Monoamine Oxidase Inhibitors* and *Tricyclic Antidepressants*, both worked on either two or all three of the neurotransmitters, not just serotonin.

*SSRIs* (or "*Selective Serotonin Re-uptake Inhibitors*") work as effective antidepressants and anti-anxiety medications by stopping your brain from recycling the serotonin you have, therefore increasing the levels floating around inside your head. In simple terms, you can think of them like the bouncer on the door of a nightclub. They let the serotonin inside but then block the exits, leading to higher levels inside.

The reasons why this helps improve the symptoms of depression and anxiety are hotly debated among scientists, as the mechanisms at work are not simple. What is clear is that it is not a simple case of - *you are low in serotonin so you just need to increase levels and you will feel better.* If this was the case, depression and anxiety would be resolved in around 3 days, the time it takes to reach full strength in your body after taking them. However, in most case, after starting *SSRI* medications, it can take up to three months before the patient feels back on track. It is clearly more complex than some pharmaceutical companies would have you believe. A more accurate statement could be that you need all of the following –

- You need the right amount of serotonin in certain parts of your brain

- You need to have the right number of serotonin receptors. An imbalance between serotonin levels and receptor functioning is clearly a potential cause of certain mental illnesses.

- You need to have enough of the substances in your diet which your body needs to make and distribute serotonin in your brain

- You need to consume enough of the building blocks of serotonin

And, most importantly –

*- You need to make sure you don't have a lifestyle or habits which perpetually deplete and keep serotonin levels low*

So, what exactly is serotonin?

Serotonin is a type of neurotransmitter - essentially a chemical that your body uses to send signals around your body and brain. So why is serotonin so important? Well, here is a quick list of some of the main aspects of your body and brain's functioning which are impacted or controlled by serotonin -

- Mood
- Anxiety
- Sleep
- Body Temperature
- Sex Drive
- Digestion

Yes, digestion! The most serotonin in your body is not in your brain, but in your gut. This is one of the reasons why anxiety and depression are usually accompanied by stomach problems like pain or poor digestion.

As you can see from the above list, if your serotonin system gets out of whack, things can get pretty unpleasant.

Now, before we move on, there are two things which you inevitably read in guides like these, particularly ones with the word *'naturally'* in the title. Firstly, you will no doubt be given the *'reason'* why serotonin deficiency *'causes'* depression or some other *'theory'* dressed up as fact. I am not going to go down this path. Anyone who claims to know exactly what causes depression and anxiety is not being truthful to you or themselves. All we have are *theories* at this stage, and the reason is, in my opinion, that everyone is different. Some people have not enough serotonin, some people too much (yes, there are drugs which alleviate depression by working the exact opposite way to *SSRIs*!), some people have a problem with dopamine, some people with noradrenaline, some people have a problem with their diet and some people have a problem with their lifestyle. Don't believe anyone who tells you *'you are depressed because of X or Y'*.

Secondly, in guides like these, you will also no doubt be told why *'antidepressant drugs are evil'* or something similar. Again, this is not the case and the situation is not black and white like some people claim. The fact is that antidepressants have helped millions of people around the world get their life back. As much as the *'natural health'* brigade have tried to claim that *SSRIs* cause brain damage, the fact is that the majority of all clinical trials and testing has shown SSRIs to actually help brains rebuild - particularly a part of the brain strongly implicated in mental illness - the *hippocampus.*

However, one thing is clear - a lot of people go on antidepressants for mild to moderate depression who don't really need to. And it is for this group of people that the evidence for antidepressants is less compelling. For mild to moderate depression, antidepressants usually don't perform any better than a *placebo* (an inert dummy pill that has no active ingredients). Coupled with the fact that antidepressants have all kinds of unpleasant side-effects, I believe that people on the milder end of the scale need to look elsewhere. And this is where this guide come in.

So why am I writing on a guide to help you increase levels of serotonin when I have just told you that there could be all kinds of causes for the way you feel? Well, in my opinion, I think serotonin is the most likely neurotransmitter to get out of whack for most people. Why is this? Again, just my opinion, however I believe various aspects of modern life are not conducive to healthy levels of serotonin. In particular, I think the high-stress, fast pace aspect of modern life sets a lot of people up for chronically low levels of serotonin.

This guide is designed to give you some relatively easy tips on either increasing levels of serotonin or maintaining the levels you have.

Before I go on, I need to stress one key point - this guide is for people mildly depressed/anxious or feeling a little below par. If you are severely depressed and particularly if you have had thoughts of self-harm, put down this book (or eBook reader!) and contact a health professional immediately. The answer to your problems will not be in this book.

Pride & Self-Esteem

Depression and anxiety, which, as I have stated, is often associated with low levels of serotonin, is commonly characterised by feelings of low self-worth or even self-loathing. Like anything in this field of study, it is difficult to ascertain the arrow of causation, meaning, is low self-esteem a cause of depression or does depression cause low self-esteem? I believe that self-esteem issues are linked back to the broader issue of social status and hierarchy. Using the primate example again, the monkeys at the bottom of the social hierarchy with low levels of serotonin are likely to be experiencing something akin to low self-esteem.

However, using the same logic we applied to the topic of socialisation, we can follow the general principle that if we 'short circuit' this process, we can lead to lasting healing. We don't know whether the urge to isolate yourself when depressed is a cause of depression (i.e. – if you had been more social in the first place, would you have developed depression?) or an effect (depression creates the urge to isolate yourself). However what we do know is that by forcing yourself to be social and have daily connections with fellow human beings, you are creating a powerful mechanism to heal yourself.

Likewise, we can apply this same principle to the feelings of low self-esteem which are associated with low levels of serotonin. What is the quickest and best way to do this? Make a concerted effort to develop feelings of pride in yourself. Naturally, you just can't force yourself to feel pride so you have to do it the old fashioned way – do things which you can be proud of our which give you a sense of achievement.

The beauty of this route to increased serotonin is that it also, as a lovely side effect, leads to increased levels of dopamine, your main pleasure and reward neurochemical.

So what are the keys to this technique?

1. Setting and achieving realistic, yet challenging goals
2. Engaging in acts of altruism and service to others

The key to goal setting is to make sure your goals are S.M.A.R.T. (Specific, Measurable, Attainable, Relevant and Time-bound)

Specific – make sure your goal is specific. Some examples of specific goals would be – finish a marathon, learn to play a certain piece of music on the piano, get a certificate of completion for a vocational course etc. The opposite of this would be vague goals like – learn to play the piano (how do you measure whether you have succeeded or not?) or practice Spanish (to what degree?)

**Measurable** – you can't track what you can't measure. Make sure you have clear measurements for success. For example, you could further refine a marathon related goal by setting a time which you need to finish the race under.
**Attainable** – make sure the goal is realistic or you will become disheartened when you can't achieve it. For example – setting the goal to lose 20 pounds in one week would not be 'attainable', however 20 pounds in 6 months would be.
**Relevant** – make sure your goal is something you are actually interested in. For example – don't set the goal of running a marathon if you have no interest whatsoever in running. Make your goal focused on something you are passionate about.
**Time-bound** – set a specific time frame. Don't make your goal open ended.

Multiple studies have shown that if you make your goals S.M.A.R.T. you are giving yourself the best possible chance for success as this type of goal setting takes into account how your brain views goals and attributes motivation accordingly. For example, to give yourself the vague goal "I want to lose weight", your brain doesn't have specific enough information to become appropriately motivated. You would need to set a weight target and a time frame.

By setting and achieving goals, you are sending a message to your subconscious that you do have things to be proud of and that you are a valuable piece of the social fabric that surrounds you. Put another way, if you are setting challenging goals and achieving them, it will become increasingly difficult for your brain to hold on to its negative self-assessment.

Something may have occurred to you at this point in my explanation – What happens if you don't achieve the goals you set? If your self-esteem does not improve through the simple act of actually working towards goals, you need to reframe your views on what is important in this whole process. Again to use the marathon example, if you get yourself to the point where you are running long distances as part of your stated goal, it becomes largely irrelevant whether you complete the race or achieve a particular time or not. You have already won the battle. To use an old quote – it's not how many times you fall over but how many times you get up again. Just by working towards your goal you have already 'picked yourself back up'.

The second path to increasing pride and self-esteem is via altruism and service. Studies have consistently shown that people who work to provide charity to others or who are motivated by a big-picture altruistic goal (such as providing meals for the homeless) are, as a group, happier than the general population. I am sure you know this instinctively. The example I always give people is to think about last time they bought something for themselves versus the last time they bought a present for another person or did something generous. It feels a lot better to give than to receive.

There are several reasons why the act of giving leads to increased levels of serotonin. Firstly, via the mechanism already stated – that selfless acts lead to a natural boost in self-esteem. I think from an evolutionary perspective, co-operation between humans has been one of our key advantages. Four people working together to bring down large prey will have more food than four people working separately, foraging for nuts and berries. Your brain has an in built circuit to reward you via increased dopamine and serotonin if you act for the good of the group, rather than for yourself only.

The other reason why this is an effective means to increase serotonin is that working towards a greater selfless cause gives your life purpose and meaning. One of the hallmarks of low serotonin (and therefore depression) is a feeling that life has no meaning or purpose. If this is you, don't sit back and wait for meaning to reveal itself to you – go out and seize it for yourself.

There is a form of Buddhist meditation called 'Loving Kindness Meditation', which involves focused, loving thoughts being held in the mind. When researchers scanned the brains of Tibetan monks doing this type of meditation, they saw levels of activity in the part of the brain involved in positive emotion, to a degree that had never previously been witnessed. Loving thoughts and loving acts are nigh on unsurpassed as paths to increased serotonin in the brain.

Increase Sun Exposure

*The Law of Unintended Consequences* says that something you had no way of predicting, always occurs as the result of a seemingly unrelated action. In this case, the unintended consequence of the *'sun smart'* message we have been taught to avoid skin cancer, has been an epidemic of low vitamin D and serotonin levels. Yes, a lack of sunlight reduces your level of serotonin.

Serotonin has strong links to sunlight which scientists are still studying to work out the exact reason why. A key link appears to be your eyes. Sunlight hitting your retina appears to tell your brain to make serotonin, however when it becomes dark, the signal to make melatonin out of serotonin is turned on. Melatonin is your body clock hormone and controls your circadian rhythm (sleep/wake cycles). Melatonin floating around your bloodstream tells your brain that it is time to sleep. As you probably guessed from the similarity in the names, melatonin and serotonin are closely related. They are like two sides of the same coin.

The best evidence of the impact on sunlight on levels of serotonin is the condition *seasonal affective disorder (SAD)*. This is a type of depression which affects people who do not get enough sun exposure in winter, particularly in cold, dark parts of the world like Canada and northern Europe. Introducing *light therapy* to sufferers, where a bright, artificial light is shone into their eyes for periods of time, raises serotonin levels and improves their mood.

Here is where this gets even more interesting. There are a group of scientists who believe that inflammation in the brain is one of the key causes of depression. One thing that has been clear for a long time is that depression is often accompanied by an increase in inflammatory conditions such as psoriasis. So this theory seems to make good sense as one of the potential causes, however you also need to bear in mind that inflammation could be the *result* of depression, not the *cause*. And what is one of the strongest ways to decrease inflammation in the body? Increase levels of vitamin D! So by giving yourself sufficient sun exposure, you are targeting depression from two angles at once - increasing levels of serotonin and decreasing inflammation.

Many scientists are calling the vitamin D deficiency epidemic the most important health crisis facing first world countries. As we cover up to avoid skin cancers, we are not giving our bodies enough chance to manufacture Vitamin D when sun hits our skin. The irony is that the majority of all deadly skin cancers are unrelated to sun exposure.

However, if you are nervous about skin cancer, there is consensus that 20 minutes of sun exposure at one time is plenty to get your vitamin D levels up and won't increase your risk of skin cancer.

Regarding serotonin, I think the best thing you can do is immediately get sunlight on your body (and directly into your eyes - meaning exposure to your eyes - please don't look directly in the sun!). By getting sunlight in your eyes when you first wake up, this not only gets serotonin flowing around your system, but also helps your body to maintain a healthy circadian rhythm.

While I am on the topic of circadian rhythm, I should also point out its importance in this area. It has been known for some time that many depressed patients appear to have a dysfunctional circadian rhythm, sending their sleep cycles haywire. Now I need to point out that why this is an important area for depressed patients is much more complicated than just serotonin. All kinds of neurochemicals and hormones are involved, such as serotonin, melatonin and cortisol. In fact, recently a new antidepressant called *agomelatine* was developed, which specifically targets melatonin and your circadian rhythm. Whilst reports on its effectiveness have been mixed, its use and effectiveness for some people clearly demonstrates a link between depression and the circadian rhythm, or at least depression and melatonin.

Meditate

Sorry to bang on so much about meditation, however If you are feeling stressed out, anxious, mildly depressed or just a little below-par, it really is a no-brainer.

Multiple studies have clearly shown that depression not only increases levels of 'feel-good' neurochemicals such as serotonin and dopamine, but also decrease levels of stress hormones such as cortisol.

In fact, in recent years, a type of therapy called "*mindfulness based stress reduction*" which involves practicing mindfulness and meditating, has become extremely popular due to its effectiveness. Now, it would be simplistic to say that this type of therapy is effective simply because of the meditation and simply because meditation increases serotonin as there are many factors at work here. However, clearly there is a beneficial link between meditation and symptoms of depression and anxiety.

The best way to think about this is to use logic. One thing is conclusive, acute and chronic stress negatively impacts your levels of serotonin. My theory is that your body uses serotonin to sooth you in times of stress, however if this becomes chronic, your body may not be able to maintain optimum levels. So what is the polar opposite of stress? That's right, meditation.

Recently I tried a little test. Despite the fact that I know they are not good for my brain, I have a little guilty pleasure which I sometimes indulge - first person shooter computer games, where you run around mowing zombies down with a shotgun. Yes I know, I should know better, but it's a nice bit of escapism every once in a while. So I decided to try something. The first day I meditated for twenty minutes and then made an assessment of my mood and physical status. After the twenty minutes I felt relaxed, blissed out a little and in a nice mood. This carried on for several hours afterward. The next day, I played my computer game for the same length of time. I had never noticed before but for some time after I was quite crabby and irritable. After playing the game, I went back to my writing and was irritated when my little boy came in and showed me something he made. All this time I had been playing these types of games and never noticed that they put me in a bad mood afterward. I have checked again several times since and found the same thing. I thought about it for a while and it makes perfect sense. These games activate your 'fight or flight system'. Certain parts of your brain are not able to discriminate between a real life zombie attack and one on your screen, so the effect on the body is the same.

Meditation, and particularly mindfulness meditation, is beneficial for serotonin levels for two reasons. Firstly, on the pure physiological level, meditation and other forms of deep relaxation, increase levels of serotonin in your brain. That is, by entering a relaxed state, you put in place the biological mechanism for increasing serotonin and decreasing stress hormones such as noradrenaline and cortisol.

The second mechanism that allows meditation to increase levels of serotonin is even more interesting. One of the aspects of mindfulness meditation is viewing your situation and your thoughts as an interested observer. So instead of the thought 'I am worthless' leading to endless rumination and a depressed mood, you just note the thought 'there I am thinking 'I am worthless''. After a while of noticing these thoughts and not reacting to them, you take the emotional sting out of them, leading to improved mood. This soon leads to the realisation that "I am not my thoughts" and this realisation gives people hope. If people (or animals) have no hope, low serotonin levels inevitably ensue (I will talk more about this later). The other key point, which I will discuss next, is that *the type of thoughts you have, impact levels of serotonin in your brain.*

Once again, for a quick and easy seated meditation technique, visit Appendix 1

## Change Your Thinking

Currently, the most common type of psychotherapy practiced in the world for anxiety and depression is called *cognitive behavioural therapy (CBT)*. CBT recognises that often mental illness is caused by faulty thinking and faulty behaviours. Regarding behaviours, I will break these up and discuss later in this guide.

The *'cognitive'* part of cognitive behavioural therapy refers to your *thinking*. One of the clearest aspects of depression is that faulty and negative thinking leads to decreased levels of serotonin. This is just an important topic that, if you think that negative or faulty thinking is a problem for you, I strongly recommend you to get some books on CBT or to visit a trained professional.

Get into the practice of being aware of the content of your thinking. Using the principles of mindfulness, just make a note of your thoughts. Over time you will start to pick up certain patterns which may be a clear cause of your low levels of serotonin. Look out for -

- Being pessimistic about the future
- Saying things in your head which feed anxiety, such as "*I am going to freak out*" or "*I won't be able to cope*"
- Making a mountain out of a molehill in your head, such as "*if I can't sleep for at least eight hours tonight I won't be able to function tomorrow*"
- Having imaginary fights with people in your head, such as imagining revenge scenarios against people you feel have wronged you
- Running negative events over and over in your head

All of the above thought patterns will, over time, decrease levels of serotonin in your brain. So, what is the opposite behaviour or thought process from the above? Practicing *'loving kindness'* and *'gratitude'*.

One of the most interesting things to come out of the collaboration between Buddhists and neuroscientists has been the practice of scanning the brains of Buddhist monks while meditating. One of the most startling findings to come out of this was that long time meditators often have a much more active *left prefrontal cortex* than the general population. The *left prefrontal cortex* is the part of the brain implicated in positive emotion. On the flip side, depressed and anxious people often show a much more active right side, the part involved in negative emotion. Further investigation has suggested that one of the best ways to achieve this effect in your head is to practice 'loving kindness' meditation. This is basically the opposite of fighting with people in your head.

Here is a simple guide to practicing loving kindness -

1. Firstly you need to develop loving kindness towards yourself. This may surprise you to hear, however poor self-esteem is often a central component of depression. So first, take some time to love yourself and forgive yourself for any past transgressions which you may feel guilty about. Remember, until you love yourself, you will be unable to love others effectively.

2. Then, start sending out loving kindness to others. I like trying easy ones first and then increasing your 'degree of difficulty', like a diving competition at the Olympics! Start with your spouse, children or other loved ones. Think about how much you love them and are grateful that they are in your life. Then, move on to neutral people. That is, those who you don't feel strongly about either way. Eventually work your way up to people you actively dislike or consider your 'enemy'. This is where the most progress is made. One technique I use, when thinking about those I dislike, is to reflect on that fact that we are all born one day and have to make our way through life the best we can. Everyone just wants to be happy and not to suffer. Purely evil sociopaths are exceedingly rare. Perhaps the person you don't like is that way because of some misfortune they have experienced?

3. There are different ways to achieve the above. You can visualise the person in your mind's eye. Visualise them smiling at you or having fun with their own loved ones. Alternatively, you can think about the positive qualities of that person or use the above technique I mentioned, thinking about how we are all the same.

A variation of loving kindness meditation is where you practice gratitude. Practicing gratitude can have almost immediate, dramatic effects on your mood and levels of serotonin. Remember, feeling hopeless or trapped by your situation leads to lower levels of serotonin, so, by extension, feeling positive and grateful about your life has the opposite effect. What people usually find is that, even though they thought their situation was hopeless and without positive aspects, after a few minutes, most people can come up with a whole heap of different things to be grateful for. Here are some suggestions on things you could be grateful for -

- Good physical health of yourself and your loved ones (naturally, not all of your loved ones will be healthy - that would be an unrealistic expectation)
- A roof over your head
- Enough food to eat
- A family that loves you
- A loving spouse
- A good job

Of course, you shouldn't look at that list and think that if you don't have one of the above points, you would have a reason to be depressed. Most people will be a mixture. For example, you could lose your job but then reflect on the fact that you have a supportive family who loves you.

So remember, positive thoughts equals more serotonin.

## Socialise

It is one of the cruellest ironies that depression leads people to cut themselves off from family and friends. Evolution usually shows a purpose for everything, however the urge to isolate yourself when depressed is one I find puzzling. Some evolutionary biologists have suggested that depression is the brain's way of telling you that something about your life or your goals is not appropriate. So your brain causes you to withdraw, giving you time to reflect on your life.

Humans are social animals and our brains are set up to reward us for socialising and integrating well with others. Social contact with family and friends is one of the strongest and most effective ways of increasing your levels of serotonin.

However, frustratingly, if you are depressed, socialising is the last thing you feel like doing. This means that you need to exert your willpower, forcing yourself to engage with others. The beauty of this is that often you will see results immediately. One minute you are feeling sorry for yourself on the couch, by yourself at home, the next you are at a dinner party with friends, laughing and connecting with others.

I can't stress this enough - one of the worst things you can do for your serotonin levels is to isolate yourself.

One of the most interesting ways to view this in action is to look at the drug *ecstasy* (MDMA), which works by dramatically increasing levels of serotonin (and to a lesser extent dopamine and noradrenaline) in your brain. Ecstasy users report an interesting phenomenon when they use the drug. When they are high (with massive levels of serotonin floating around their brain), there is an overpowering urge to socialise and connect with people. Users report that the simple act of meeting up with a friend while high, sends their serotonin levels through the roof, giving them rushes of pleasure. Now I am not about to recommend anyone try this (nothing depletes serotonin quicker than MDMA), however by showing the extremes of what serotonin does in your brain, it provides some useful information. MDMA exaggerates everything, so while you don't get *'rushes of pleasure'* when you socialise while not on the drug, there is definitely a positive effect on serotonin. Interestingly, when users have crashed after using MDMA, they report the opposite. They enter a 'mini-depression' where they can't bear the thought of socialising.

If you are depressed, it probably won't be easy at first, however you simply must force yourself to socialise. If necessary, start easy - maybe just a phone call to a friend or relative or a quick coffee with a friend. Slowly you can then work your way up to a night on the town or a dinner party. It will be worth it. Your serotonin receptors will thank you for it!

## Massage

Multiple studies have also shown that massage decreases the stress hormone cortisol while increasing levels of serotonin and dopamine. Again the reasons behind this are not completely clear yet, however one thing is well known to science - the impact on human touch to other humans.

There was a famous case involving Romanian orphans after the fall of the communist dictatorship there at the end of the 1980s. Due to neglect, the orphans at a particular orphanage had not received any human touch. These orphans displayed all kinds of psychological and physical impairments from the lack of human contact. They had dysfunctional cortisol systems due to the chronic stress of receiving no human contact.

Human beings are designed to touch and be touched. This can be at the sexual level or at the level of a mother hugging her baby.

Touching or being touched leads to increased levels of serotonin and one of the best ways to do this is via massage.

The beauty of massage is that even someone who is isolated can visit a masseuse and receive massage therapy for a fee. This is vitally important for someone without a partner who is depressed or lonely.

Full body oil massages in particular can be very effective as they maximise the skin contact between masseuse and the recipient. Massage works from two angles at once. It decreases stress hormones and increases serotonin. Plus, if you get some deep tissue work, it can also eliminate the physical manifestations of stress which are held in tight muscles.

## Avoid alcohol

Yes, sorry – alcohol. *Again!*

It is a testament to the addictive nature of alcohol consumption that when I lay out all the ways for people to get their serotonin levels up, the main one which I get resistance on is the consumption of alcohol. Regular and heavy consumers of alcohol have no idea that they are completely addicted to it, just like a heroin addict is with heroin. It is the very definition of an addiction when people cannot give it up even when they know it is harmful for them.

For the average person who is not under a lot of stress and with the low levels of serotonin which come with this, the odd glass of wine or beer is not really going to be any problem. However, for someone with low serotonin levels, alcohol can be a massive problem for several reasons.

Firstly, alcohol gives you a nice short term boost in your serotonin levels. This is one of the reasons why doctors believe that the majority of alcoholism cases are really just self-medicating for depression. Someone who has been depressed for a long time due to low serotonin reasons, as an example, has slowly realised over time that with that first glass of alcohol comes sweet relief from their depression, due to the bump in serotonin they get. Then, as their serotonin levels dip after the first glass, they have more and more to keep chasing that relief. Alcohol plays havoc with your serotonin system so should be avoided for this reason.

Along with this, there is another problem with alcohol - it completely messes up your sleep quality. You know that tired and depressed feeling you get the day after drinking too much? That is an exaggerated effect of what alcohol consumption does to your sleep. Alcohol prevents you from getting enough of your most important stages of sleep - *Slow Wave Sleep* (deep sleep) and *REM sleep* (rapid eye movement). You spend most of the night in light sleep. Why is this a problem apart from the fact you feel bad? Deep sleep is where your brain replenishes your hormones and neurotransmitters. Deprive yourself of this stage and you are not allowing your brain to get its serotonin levels back on track. And if you are already depressed, this can be particularly concerning. Depression is associated with too much REM and light sleep and not enough Slow Wave Sleep. You are exaggerating this existing problem by consuming alcohol.

Furthermore, by drinking alcohol to escape the way you feel, you are training your brain to believe that this is the only way you can make yourself feel better. By developing coping mechanisms that come from within, you are sending the message to your subconscious that you have the power to heal yourself. This sense of control is a nice segway into the next one on my list.

## Fight or Flight?

One of the classic behavioural experiments involving those poor unfortunate mice, gives us great insight into the way the mind works. If you put a mouse into an environment where it gets electric shocks and has no way to escape or control the situation, its serotonin levels plummet and it exhibits all the symptoms of depression. Similarly, scientists have found that serotonin levels are much higher in primates who are the 'alpha dog' in their group, compared to the ones lower down the chain. The key is hope and control.

If you feel trapped, with a lack of control over your situation, serotonin levels will decrease accordingly. This can mean an abusive relationship or a dead end job you hate. If your brain senses that you have no control, serotonin levels will drop. So to combine the above two situations with the mice and the monkeys, the worst possible situation is for you to be in a job you hate, where you are at the bottom of the food chain. This is a dangerous recipe for low serotonin.

You need to take back control. If your job is a problem, start making a plan on how to fix the situation (serotonin and dopamine levels increase when you make realistic plans to alleviate any unpleasant situation). This may mean - starting some new study to gain new skills, plotting how to get a promotion to a better job in your existing company or proactively looking for a better job. If you are depressed and your financial situation allows it, don't hesitate to quit your job to then take stock of where you are at. Never, ever put your career ahead of your health.

Think about the mice or the downtrodden monkeys. Does your subconscious view your current circumstance in the same way? If so, take action immediately.

However, does this advice depend on whether we are anxious, or depressed? I think it may, and I only had this realisation recently.

I read a LOT of research papers on the brain. In fact, it's one of the best ways I get a restful sleep. Just lay in bed with a paper on the atrophy of the rat hippocampus and I am guaranteed to be sound asleep within minutes. Recently I was reading a paper when I had the most interesting realization – and it was only because of the fact that I read two different papers in short succession that enabled me to realise something dramatic and important for those suffering anxiety or depression.

The first paper I read discussed the fact that avoidance of whatever you are afraid of, only increases the fear. If you suffer anxiety and have had some form of psychotherapy, this would be nothing new. You will often hear the expression "A fear avoided is a fear doubled" in the area of treating anxiety disorders. For example, if you are afraid of flying and therefore avoid ever going on an aeroplane, you are sending a clear message to your sub-conscious that flying IS dangerous and needs to be avoided. Your subconscious (specifically, your amygdala) will respond by increasing the warning signals whenever this feared event looms. This is where Exposure Therapy comes in. With Exposure Therapy, you are gradually exposed to the feared event in small doses, so over time, your brain will slowly start to relax in response to the event. For example, if you are afraid of spiders, you will be shown a photo of a spider, followed by real spider and then perhaps finishing with holding a (non-venomous) spider in your hand.

Next I read a paper on mice and serotonin. In this paper, researchers demonstrated how, when you place a mouse in a stressful situation with no sense of control or hope of escape, serotonin levels drop and they display the hallmarks of depression. This logic can then be extended to humans. As I mentioned in the previous section, if you are in a hopeless and stressful situation with no hope of escape, depression is a likely outcome.

After reading these two papers I suddenly realised that they were indirectly recommending the opposite thing. One suggested that you need to stay and confront whatever it is that is stressing you or making you afraid, while the other suggested the need to have a sense of hope or ability to escape an unpleasant situation.

You MUST spend some time to gain insight into your current situation to determine whether FIGHT (stay and confront your fears or the source of your distress) or FLIGHT (escape your current situation) is appropriate. If I was forced to simplify, I would say that if you are on the anxious spectrum and have no depressive symptoms, you should confront your fears. If you are on the depressive spectrum, you need to escape or at least create a means of possible escape. However, remember that this is a simplification and is likely to be more complex than just "anxious" or "depressed".

If you decided that escape is your best course of action, don't let anyone tell you that you are 'running away from your problems'. There are good ways and bad ways to do this. Think about it in terms of military strategy – you are beating a strategic retreat to enable you to fight another battle on another front.

In evolutionary terms, one of the theories of depression is that it developed as a way of telling an animal that something about its current predicament is not beneficial. Depression therefore causes the animal (or human) to lose motivation and withdraw to consider its situation. Unfortunately, almost every aspect of the human body has evolved to overreact to everything, because, over millions of years, overreacting gives more chance of survival than underreacting. It's why the body goes into full panic mode at the slightest hint of a bacterial or viral invader. Unfortunately, this also holds true for some people with depression. The brain has had such a strong reaction to an unacceptable situation that some people are unable to get back on their feet again.

If you are depressed, often it is your brain trying to tell you that you need to escape your current situation. You need to consider whether you are just the human equivalent of a little mouse getting electric shocks inside of a box they can't escape.

The sense of feeling trapped in a particular situation is one of the main triggers for suicide attempts. A person is trapped by financial hardship, violence or disgrace and feels like there is no hope of escape. This is why I believe that you need to gain a clear sense of what exactly is causing your current mood problems and act accordingly.

It is rare that any situation is genuinely inescapable. Of course there are some situations where escape, in the physical sense, is impossible – such as when someone is jailed or held captive – however these situations are rare.

In those rare situations where escape is actually not possible, I believe you need to reframe your definition of 'escape'. The way you do this is by reframing the situation as a positive in some way. For example, being jailed can be used as a time for reflection or learning a new skill.

Here is the process I recommend you following –

1. Am I anxious or depressed?
2. If I am anxious but not depressed, I need to focus on facing my fears to extinguish my anxiety
3. If I am depressed, I need to identify what exactly it is about my current situation that is causing me to feel trapped or without hope
4. Formulate a plan for escaping my current situation in a productive way. For example, if you are trapped in a dead-end or stressful job you hate, start studying a new skill. This sends a subtle signal to your brain that you have options
5. If escape (under your current definition) is not possible, reframe your definition of 'escape' to again send a signal to your brain that you have control over the situation. To use the prison example again, if you spend every day in jail distressed that you are trapped, you will surely become depressed. However, if you reframe it as an opportunity to learn accounting or how to paint, you have escaped your predicament to an extent, as far as your subconscious mind is concerned.

## Reduce Sources of Stress

So now that you have started meditating, you have an important tool to deal with stress. You have a fire extinguisher to put out the fire.

However, don't you think you should also work to *stop lighting so many fires*?

Stress is the biggest enemy of serotonin that there is. A chronically stressed individual will not have a lot of this feel good chemical floating around their brain.

You need to make a brutal assessment of all the sources of stress in your life and then work to reduce or eliminate them. Some common sources of stress -

- Money troubles
- Taking on too many responsibilities and feeling like you cannot cope
- Frequent fighting with your partner or spouse
- Serious health problems of someone close to you
- A job with more things to do than hours in the day
- A job which involves regular conflict

Some sources of stress are unavoidable. We will come to those in a minute. For the sources of stress which are avoidable, you need to be brutal and eliminate them from your life. Say no to that request to join another committee. Say no to that extra work your co-worker tries to dump on you because you usually don't complain. Get out of a poisonous relationship.

Regarding the sources of stress which are unavoidable, first you need to use some of the techniques in this guide such as meditation, to reduce your reaction to the stress. There is a great quote "*In life there will be waves so you'd better grab a surfboard.*" This is saying that often there is no way to avoid stress, so you need to find ways to cope with it better. Often this involves reframing the situation from a negative to a positive. Perhaps you use financial troubles to prompt you to look at a change of careers that could lead to you discovering your passion. Perhaps the health problems of a loved one help you to appreciate them and you can view the situation as a lesson on appreciating people while they are around. Whatever you have to do to reframe the situation from a stress-provoking one to a positive or neutral one.

## Engage in Repetitive Behaviour

Here is another one of those strange ones I found buried in a couple of research papers that you never hear of – engaging in repetitive behaviours increases levels of serotonin.

If you watch certain animals, they often do certain things over and over. A good example is a cat or a dog that licks itself over and over. How many times have you watched your pet and said "Surely that's enough – looks pretty clean to me!"

This also applies to humans. It has long been known that Obsessive Compulsive Disorder (OCD) is often characterised by low levels of serotonin in the sufferer's brain. It has been theorised that the repetitive behaviours seen in OCD may be a subconscious way of increasing levels of serotonin and relieving some of the distress. You often also see this in some autistic children, who, when distressed, will retreat somewhere safe and engage in something repetitive like flicking a light switch off and on.

I believe that at least some of the pleasure of running and jogging comes from the repetitive nature of it. I have always believe that the 'runner's high' comes more from serotonin than from endorphins. This was recently proven in an experiment where runners were given a drug which blocks the action of pain receptors. The runners still experienced the same good feeling, which means that 'runner's high' is not fully explained by endorphins.

Interestingly, in the study I read, chewing gum was mentioned as a quick and easy way to increase serotonin via a repetitive action. Unfortunately I haven't been able to test this out myself as chewing gum gives me a sore jaw.

When studying serotonin, I often look to studies on users of the drug ecstasy, as this is an example of people with extremely high levels of serotonin (at least until they crash that is). What immediately stuck out to me is the fact that ecstasy users love dancing to repetitive, tribal techno music as it increases the high. And what else do almost all ecstasy users love to do while high? That's right, chew gum.

There is some connection with chewing and serotonin that I have not yet been able to ascertain. High levels of serotonin (whether by SSRI medications or ecstasy) is often associated with jaw clenching and repetitive jaw movements. However in the meantime, it does appear clear that chewing, and other repetitive movements, increase levels of serotonin in the brain. Your challenge now is to find some kind of repetitive movement that you enjoy and can maintain.

Supplements that increase serotonin

I have to admit that I am a little torn as to whether I should include supplements in this list of ways to increase your serotonin. There are several reasons for this.

Firstly, there is an inherent problem with taking a pill to increase serotonin. As opposed to the other methods in this guide, it does not involve any effort whatsoever on your part. If we think back to the concept of *effort based rewards*, we realise that we are not helping our neurochemistry by engaging in something effortful that results in higher levels of serotonin and dopamine. Also we are sending a message to our subconscious that the answer to the problem lies outside of us, in a pill. I think that this is not helpful in the long run, as developing your own strategies to increase serotonin through your own efforts is a much better long term proposition.

Secondly, the line between 'pharmaceuticals' and 'supplements' (or 'natural') is grey. People are often deluded that 'natural' equals 'gentle' or 'safe', when often this is not the case. Also you need to use your powers of common sense. When you hear that an herb increases serotonin, how do you think it achieves it? Yes, you guessed it, by the same ways that pharmaceuticals do in most cases. For example, the majority of all herbs used to increase serotonin, do it by acting either as an SSRI or as a Monoamine Oxidase Inhibitor - just like the drugs do.

That said, there are a few supplements out there which increase serotonin in a much milder way than drugs and with fewer side effects. So if you think that you need a little help on top of the techniques already mentioned in this guide, feel free to investigate the following supplements. However, please keep in mind that even the best 'natural' antidepressant is going to have only a fraction of the effectiveness of a 'pharmaceutical' antidepressant for more severe cases of mood dysfunction. Therefore I can really only recommend them for the mildest of cases. That said, if we are talking a 'mild' case of anxiety or depression, some of the 'natural' options are much better than the SSRIs. Remember, taking SSRIs is a big decision and should only be done if you make the decision you cannot cope without their assistance. There are big downsides to SSRIs (such as sexual dysfunction, weight gain etc.) which are only tolerable in comparison to the alternative – staying anxious or depressed. If you are seriously ill, don't mess around with Bach Flower Essences or similar hocus pocus, get to your doctor and get on something pharmaceutical.

## St. John's Wort

This is the gold standard of herbal antidepressants for a good reason - in cases of mild to moderate depression, it has been shown in multiple clinical studies to work just as well as drugs. There is debate as to whether it functions as an SSRI or as a Monoamine Oxidase Inhibitor, however this is irrelevant. What is important is whether it works or not. One of the most impressive aspects of SJW is that in one study it outperformed SSRIs in terms of increasing levels of BDNF. The main problem with St John's Wort (and it is a big problem), is that it interacts with a huge list of other medicines. Essentially, it affects how your body metabolises other medicines, which can cause problems when it stops them from working. My general rule is that if you are taking any kind of medicine at all, give St John's Wort a miss.

## Rhodiola Rosea

In my opinion, this can often be a better option than St John's Wort as there are fewer interactions with other medications. Rhodiola functions as a Monoamine Oxidase Inhibitor, which means it also raises levels of dopamine and noradrenaline, not just serotonin. So if you have problems with high levels of dopamine and/or noradrenaline, you might need to give this one a miss and concentrate on something which works more purely on serotonin. As a bonus, this herb has been used for many years to heal the brain after a period of high stress. It is classed as an 'adaptogen', a class of herbs which I am in general suspicious about. Adaptogens are supposed to 'support' the body in vague, non-specific ways that naturopaths love to exploit. If you are stressed, adaptogens supposedly calm you down; if you don't have enough energy, they give you energy. There is no such thing as a free lunch in pharmacology, so adaptogens in general have earned my scorn. However, rhodiola is one which has stood up to various trials and appears to work as a pretty decent antidepressant. For some people it can even be quite stimulating so you may need to avoid taking it after lunch.

## Inositol

This is a substance usually found in B-Group Vitamin supplements and synthesized in the body from glucose. Inositol plays a vital role in the modulation of serotonin activity in the brain and has been extensively studied as an antidepressant. It has been shown to be an effective treatment (in high enough doses) for anxiety, depression and obsessive compulsive disorder (OCD).

## SAM-e

SAM-e is another popular antidepressant alternative which may be worth investigating. As I mentioned at the start of the guide, depression is caused by all kinds of different things. SAM-e addresses one part of your brain's activity and if this part (called *Methyl Group Transfers* for those interested in looking into it in more detail) is dysfunctional, you may get some benefit. The exact mechanism of action is unclear however it is believed that for some people, a shortage of SAM-e in the system can cause problems with the synthesis of neurotransmitters such as serotonin. A bonus of SAM-e is that it has also been shown to improve symptoms of arthritis. The major downside is that it is expensive. A cheaper alternative is to supplement with Trimethylglycine ("TMG"), which is believed to have similar effects as SAM-e supplementation.

## L-Methylfolate

Folate is an important co-factor in the production of serotonin in your brain. In many studies, folate supplementation led to increased levels of serotonin (or the metabolites of serotonin) in the spinal fluid of depressed subjects. However, a certain percentage of the population is unable to convert folic acid into L-Methylfolate inside their body, leading to lower levels of serotonin. There is now even a pharmaceutical version of L-Methylfolate available which is sometimes given to patients who do not respond to SSRI medications (if you can't do this conversion in your body, you will not be able to derive any benefit from SSRIs). Therefore, I think the best option would be to supplement with L-Methylfolate instead of straight folic acid

## Curcumin

I believe curcumin is something that a lot of people should be supplementing with, even if they do not suspect that they have low levels of serotonin. Curcumin is derived from turmeric, the ingredient used in Indian curries. Curcumin is not only a potent anti-inflammatory but has also been shown to protect against some forms of cancer. As well as its anti-inflammatory action, it has a beneficial effect on serotonin levels via its action as a weak monoamine oxidase inhibitor.

## B6

B6 is, like folate, an important B-Group vitamin used in the production of serotonin. If you are deficient in B6, you will most likely be deficient in serotonin. B-Group vitamins are water-soluble, which means we need to consume them regularly because our body does not store them. Therefore I recommend a B-Group multivitamin which has all the different B-Group vitamins.

### Tryptophan/5-htp

Serotonin is called a '*monoamine*', which means that it is manufactured by a single amino acid and in the case of serotonin, this amino acid is called L-tryptophan and is contained in all kinds of foods like meat and bananas, for example. The process goes - L-tryptophan => 5-htp => serotonin. So if you are deficient in the amino acid building blocks through your dietary intake, you may have a problem with insufficient serotonin. There is some controversy around how effective it is to consume Tryptophan or 5-htp to increase serotonin levels, however it could be worth a try. Many people swear by 5-htp in particular.

### Omega 3 Fatty Acids

Another supplement that we all should be taking, low serotonin or not, is omega 3 Fatty Acids. You have probably heard about this type of fat, found mainly in seafood, which is good for your heart and your brain. What you probably haven't heard is that these fats have been used as effective treatments for both standard depression and also for bi-polar depression. As to why these fats improve depression is a little less clear. One of the strongest theories is that omega 3 Fatty Acids improve the permeability of cell membranes (how easy molecules can travel through the cell walls), leading to an improved ability for serotonin to travel to where it is needed in the brain.

# Chapter 4 – Jump-start your brain with exercise

For those of you who are familiar with my other books and guides, I like to cut out all the waffle and get straight to the point, so let me get straight to the point of this guide –

*Study after study has clearly shown that cardiovascular exercise and/or weight training works just as well as antidepressant medication, but with one key advantage - Those subjects who treat their anxiety and depression with exercise tend to stay well, whereas those who treat their depression with medication have a significantly higher relapse rate.*

And this is not just fringe research. This is mainstream research by reputable universities and scientific organisations, reported in renowned scientific journals. Whether you refer to the *Mayo Clinic* or the *Black Dog Institute*, all will recommend exercise therapy as a first-line tool to treat depression (*Note - from the point on, unless there is a distinction, I will stick to the term "depression" when referring generally to mood disorders such as major depressive disorder, atypical depression or generalized anxiety disorder*).

So if the evidence is so clear-cut, why isn't exercise recommended as the first treatment option by the majority of doctors? There are a variety of reasons, including –

- **Habit** - Doctors are risk-averse and like to stick to what works. This is particularly the case for serious conditions such as heart disease, cancer and depression. Just like doctors will continue to prescribe statins despite the lack of efficacy for preventing heart attacks (unless you fit a particular high-risk group), they will continue to focus on pharmacotherapy for depression. They are keenly aware that severely depressed patients are at risk of suicide, so they will want to do what they know has worked in the past as the death of a patient weighs heavily on the mind of any physician.

- **Legal Liability** - Any time a doctor does anything which doesn't conform to what is currently "standard practice", if something happens to the patient, they potentially open themselves up to legal liability. Again to use statins as an example - Currently statins are the "standard practice" if someone has high-cholesterol numbers. The research tells us that for this group of people (high cholesterol but no previous heart attack or evidence of heart disease)at best statins would only prevent 2 heart attacks for every 100 people. However, if a doctor doesn't prescribe statins and someone has a heart attack (which, statistically, is going to happen, whether they are on statins or not), the doctor is potentially open to legal action. Or, put another way - the data also tells us that, of those 100 people taking statins, 4 are at an increased risk for diabetes and cognitive dysfunction. However, because a doctor is following accepted practice, they are at little risk for being sued if a patient develops diabetes from taking statins. Similarly, a doctor is unlikely to be at risk of legal action if they prescribe medication and a patient commits suicide.

- **Medication tends to work more quickly than exercise therapy** - Benefits of antidepressants tend to start emerging around the 4 week point, with exercise and Cognitive Behavioral Therapy (CBT) a little while after. If a doctor is worried about the severity of depression, they may want to act more aggressively to knock it on the head as soon as possible. However, this must also be balanced against the fact that often antidepressant treatment is associated with a temporary worsening of depression when first started. This is the period when the severely depressed are most at risk of suicide.

However, by far the main reason why exercise therapy is not the first line of treatment is also the most powerful theme of this guide and also the reason why the effects tend to last - Starting an exercise program while you are depressed is seriously tough sometimes. It can seem like a superhuman effort is required and some people just can't muster the willpower. Remember - this is not a reflection on these people as the very illness they need willpower to beat, also happens to sap their willpower. However, and this is a big "however", *this is also the reason why the effects tend to last.* You give yourself a sense of achievement by getting out of bed or off the sofa and onto the track or into the gym. And here is the key point which I would like you to think about for a moment - *You have conquered depression through your own effort, not from a pill bottle.*

Renowned psychologist and author Martin Seligman (Author of "*Authentic Happiness*") has popularized the term *learned optimism*, which is the diametrical opposite to *learned helplessness*, a state highly associated with depression. So what does *learned helplessness* mean? It refers to the loss of control over a person's (or animal's) life which often triggers depression. When researchers study those poor old mice, they consistently notice something extremely interesting. When you take away an animal's control over their environment (usually by giving them small electric shocks which they cannot stop or control), they soon start exhibiting signs of depression.

So, by starting an exercise program while depressed, you are taking back control over your environment and situation. This is incredibly important for your brain and for your subconscious mind.

As with my other guides, such as Increase Serotonin Naturally, the aim of this guide is to distill all the research and background information into an easy to read, quick-reference guide which covers -

- *What does the research say?*
- *How exactly does exercise treat depression?*
- *How to put it into practice*

Remember to be gentle with yourself. If you don't feel up to this just yet, don't beat yourself up about it. I often refer to antidepressants as *training wheels*, which help you to get back on your bike again without the risk of falling and hurting yourself. Using this analogy, it's perfectly fine to use the strategy of starting antidepressants to give you that first initial spark which gives you the energy to start exercising. Then, as the benefits of exercise start accruing, with your doctor's permission, you can perhaps look to start slowly tapering off your medication (For more information on how to come off medication with as little difficulty as possible, please refer to my book Quitting *Antidepressants the Easy Way - A Guide to Stopping Medications for Anxiety and Depression).*

When deciding on a strategy for treating any illness you might have, the first question you should ask yourself every time is - *What does the research say?*

If something is not verified in research studies, it is just an opinion or an anecdote. Anecdotes are incredibly dangerous because we as humans have very poor abilities to ignore isolated cases when forming opinions. Let me give you an example - Say you have had been experiencing stomach aches for months and doctors are unable to give you a diagnosis or perhaps you receive a general diagnosis of irritable bowel syndrome (IBS) as they cannot find anything physically wrong with you. In this scenario, most people will then try a variety of medications and supplements to try to get rid of their stomach ache. Then, one day your stomach aches happen to disappear on the exact same day that you took a large dose of vitamin C. If you are a typical person, you will surely feel confident that the vitamin C cured your stomach aches, right? I am also betting that just now when I posed this question to you, you were confident in your ability to ignore this as a possible co-incidence right? So, say that you tell your friends about your stomach aches stopping after taking vitamin C and they also try it. Slowly, over time, this hypothesis may get widespread attention, and here's where the research comes in.

Scientists can then test the vitamin c/stomach ache hypothesis with a *double-blind, placebo-controlled trial.* In trials like these, a group of patients (say, 100 people) will be split into two groups. In this case, it would be - 50 people taking vitamin C and 50 people taking a placebo (an inert sugar pill usually). They key points are –

- Each patient has no idea which group he is in
- The people giving out the pills have no idea which pills they are giving

Then, at the end of the trial, the data is compiled to see if the group taking the vitamin C saw any statistically significant benefit. By "statistically significant", it means that if, for example, the vitamin C group had one more person get better than the placebo group it is not considered enough to prove any benefit. There needs to be a clear pattern of benefit in the vitamin C group.

These kinds of trials cut through any personal biases and distortions. So, when you want to find out if something works, your first step should be reviewing any research on whatever it is you are studying.

However, there is another complication. Say for example that there are 100 different studies around the world on vitamin C for stomach aches. Statistical probability says that, even by pure chance, at least one or two of these studies may show that vitamin C cures stomach aches. This is where *meta-analyses* come in. Meta-analyses pool together all the different studies to create one big study that has much better statistical grounding. In general, if a meta-analysis is positive, scientists are fairly certain that the result correctly reflects reality.

So, that leads us on to the most recent meta-analysis looking at exercise for depression, which was conducted by the University of Toronto's George Mammen and published in the *American Journal of Preventive Medicine*. In his study, Mammen, along with Professor Guy Faulkner, looked at a massive pool of over 26 years' of research and found a strong, clear link between increased exercise and a lessening of depressive symptoms. They applied a strict criteria for including any study in their analysis, to ensure that the conclusions reached would be robust. In the end, they whittled a massive number of trials and citations down to 30 individual studies. Of these, 25 showed a clear and consistent benefit of exercise for depression.

Interestingly, Mammen and Faulkner also found that you didn't need to necessarily engage in high-intensity exercise to see any benefit. Even low-intensity activity such as walking or gardening was associated with an improvement in symptoms. For Mammen, the results were clear *"It's definitely worth taking note that if you're currently active, you should sustain it. If you're not physically active, you should initiate the habit. This review shows promising evidence that the impact of being active goes far beyond the physical."*

In another single study (not a meta-analysis) by Duke University Neuroscientist James Blumenthal, which was published in the Archives of Internal Medicine, 156 people with depression were broken up into three groups. The first group did aerobic exercise, the second group took the antidepressant Zoloft (sertraline) and the third group did a combination of both. After four months, more than two-thirds of all subjects were no longer considered to be depressed. The differences between the groups was sufficiently minor that the organizers were confident in concluding that exercise appeared to have similar efficacy to antidepressants. However, importantly, there were two key points to bear in mind. Firstly, the groups receiving the Zoloft saw benefit a little earlier than the group doing exercise only, so medication appears to have a possible advantage in terms of speed of remission. However this needs to be balanced against the possible increase in suicide risk early in antidepressant treatment. The second key point only emerged when the study organizers followed up with the subjects later and found that the patients who continued to exercise were less likely to have become depressed again in the interim. Of the group taking medication in the study, 38% had relapsed into depression, whereas among the exercise group, only 8% had relapsed! Regarding the reason for this large difference, Blumenthal said *"One of the positive psychological benefits of systematic exercise is the development of a sense of personal mastery and positive self-regard, which we believe is likely to play some role in the depression-reducing effects of exercise"*.

In another meta-analysis which was only recently updated, the Cochrane Corporation conducted a similar study to that conducted by George Mammen and Guy Faulkner, looking at 35 trials' worth of data on exercise as a treatment for depression. The authors of this study reached roughly the same conclusion as the other analysis however couched the results in more cautious or neutral terminology. The authors concluded *"Exercise is moderately more effective than a control intervention for reducing symptoms of depression, but analysis of methodologically robust trials only shows a smaller effect in favor of exercise…When compared to psychological or pharmacological therapies, exercise appears to be no more effective, though this conclusion is based on a few small trials."* So, while it is possible to say clearly that exercise has roughly the same benefit as antidepressants or psychotherapy, in the context of a study, no single option has a clear demonstrable advantage. Unfortunately this Cochrane review did not mention follow-up study, which is where the most interesting aspect of this discussion tends to emerge - the apparent advantage of exercise in the longer term.

I think we are now at a stage where the benefits of exercise have been consistently demonstrated in study after study, so the only debate remaining is around the degree of benefit. As mentioned, we are not talking about niche studies in unheard of journals. Even the renowned Nurses' Health Study, which tracked around 50,000 women, showed that active women showed much lower rates of depression than sedentary counterparts.

Put simply, study after study has demonstrated several consistent effects of exercise for mood disorders –

- There is a clear association between levels of physical activity and rates of depression. As activity levels decrease, anxiety and depression increase. This demonstrates the powerful benefits of exercise as a *preventative* for mood disorders.
- Once someone has become depressed or developed an anxiety disorder, exercise performs in a roughly equivalent fashion to antidepressant medication in *treating* the illness.
- Once a mood disorder has been treated by either exercise or medication, those that used exercise to treat their illness were dramatically less likely to relapse.

If exercise were a drug and you assessed it solely on the benefits versus the risk profile or side-effect profile, it would be the dominant antidepressant in the world today. In fact, exercise is not only free of the side-effects seen with SSRI drugs (such as Prozac, Zoloft etc.), it actually improves your sex life via increased levels of dopamine and better blood flow. I had a client (who will remain anonymous for obvious reasons) who, for reasons unknown to me, occasionally measured the length of his penis. After starting an exercise program he discovered a strange effect that I had never read of before – his penis grew by around half an inch! He attributed this to the improved blood flow which accompanies a great degree of physical fitness. I have no idea whether this is a widespread phenomenon and I have no idea whether you would be able to replicate it (if you are male, naturally), but it is an interesting report nonetheless.

So, if we are to accept that there is an undeniable benefit, the natural follow up question should be - *how does it work?*

How does exercise treat depression?

I think the fact that exercise clearly works as a treatment for mood disorders is a much more important point than *how* it works. Remember that there are a range of medications that we know work, despite the mechanism being poorly understood. For example, you might be surprised to know that while we know acetaminophen (paracetamol) works to treat mild pain, exactly how it works is still the subject of some debate. In contrast, we clearly know how opiates work (as opiate receptor agonists) and how ibuprofen works (by reducing inflammation), whereas acetaminophen is a little less clear.

Similarly, there is considerable debate among scientists as to exactly how exercise works to treat depression. As I mentioned, this doesn't particularly concern me apart for one small point. If further research can shed light on the true mechanism (or more likely, mechanisms) behind the effects of exercise on mood, it may enable us to tailor exercise programs specifically for depressed patients.

At present, the main hypotheses are -

### 1. The "Endorphin" Theory
This theory is probably the most widely known. It says that strenuous exercise causes a spike in endorphins which makes you feel good. Endorphins are like your body's own natural morphine - hence the name "endorphin" being derived from "endogenous morphine". When you stub your toe or do something equally painful, you may have noticed a moment of blinding pain followed by a sudden decrease in pain and a vaguely pleasurable sensation. You have endorphins to thank for this.

For many years scientists wondered why the human brain and body would have receptors that appeared to be designed perfectly for morphine. Why would your body have a special design to obtain pain relief from juice extracted from an obscure plant that only grew naturally in small parts of the world (the opium poppy)? Then researchers discovered that we are able to make our own morphine as a way to soothe pain.

However, while many people know that endorphins and morphine kill physical pain, most people don't realise that they also soothe psychological pain. Herein lies the danger of opiate drugs. If opiates like heroin or oxycodone only treated physical pain, they would not be so psychologically addictive. This is also one of the reasons why becoming addicted to opiate drugs is strongly associated with traumatic and stressful environments. Opiates are the strongest possible way to soothe stress. When someone in a difficult life situation gets high on heroin, all their troubles melt away.

Unfortunately, opiate addicts can also show us what happens when things go wrong with your opiate and endorphin system in your brain. One thing which scientists have known for a long time is that long term heroin addicts have extremely poor stress tolerance. The slightest stressor can be unbearable for an addict (when they are not high). It is believed that this is because, after years of having heroin do all the work soothing stress, the brain of an addict slowly loses the ability to do it without the assistance of heroin. Their endorphin system down-regulates.

There is a theory regarding a similar, but slightly different phenomenon at work in the brain of someone depressed or anxious - particularly if chronic, long-term stress is the cause of the mood disorder. Another thing which researchers have noticed is that children who experience chronic stress have a dramatically higher chance of developing a mood disorder later in life. Linked to this is another interesting phenomenon - fibromyalgia.

Fibromyalgia is a pain disorder where the sufferer experiences a range of debilitating symptoms but with the primary symptom being chronic pain with no physical cause (like an injury or inflammation). One of the most common triggers for fibromyalgia is a period of extreme stress. A prominent theory is that, after putting your body's endorphin and opiate system under such massive strain, something eventually "breaks", leading to chronic pain. It is thought that there may be a problem with either actual endorphins or the receptors that endorphins are supposed to activate. To use an oversimplified analogy, it is possible that intolerable amounts of stress leads to chronically high levels of endorphins (to deal with the stress), which means that over time, the same receptors need more and more endorphins just to activate. This is a similar theory behind why it can take time for your brain to adjust after taking antidepressants - your receptors get lazy as they don't have to work hard to get the serotonin (because there is more floating around in the synapses).

So, if we accept the theory that depression (and similar conditions such as fibromyalgia) are associated with endorphin or opiate receptor dysfunction, the logical question is - how do we rectify the situation? That's where exercise comes in.

I bet you have heard of the "runner's high", where, after a period of strenuous exercise, you start to feel strangely peaceful, pain-free and even euphoric. It has long been theorized that this is due to your endorphins kicking in, with evolution giving you a little helping hand to get you past the pain. From an evolutionary perspective this makes perfect sense. Throughout human history, strenuous exercise like sprinting or running long distances is associated with either trying to catch your dinner or trying to avoid becoming another creature's dinner. If your endorphins give you a second wind, it can be the difference between life and death.

So, the endorphin theory says that by exercising, the depressed person gets a boost in endorphins, making them feel better. And if this is repeated regularly, there will be a gradual improvement in how the person feels on a day to day basis and therefore mood will naturally improve.

This effect has even been verified in well-constructed studies such as the one by Boecker et al which was published in the journal *Cerebral Cortex*. In this study, a substance was used which allows researchers to see what is happening in different parts of the brain of 10 athletes. The athletes were scanned initially to get a baseline reading, before being sent on a 2 hour run (I hope they were paid well!). This trial clearly showed that exercise increased endorphin activity in areas of the brain associated with euphoria and positive mood.

However, here is where things get a little more complicated. In other study by Janal et al, subjects were given a drug called *nalaxone*. Nalaxone is a drug which negates the effects of any opiate - it is given to people who have overdosed on heroin to keep them alive. What these researchers found was that nalaxone negated the euphoric effects of "runner's high" but not the other effects such as pain relief and how "co-operative" the subject were. This suggests that, while endorphins may be an important component of how exercise helps depression, they are not the whole picture. Which leads us to the second theory.

## 2. The "Monoamine" Theory
Interestingly, the neurotransmitter most associated with levels of co-operation is serotonin, which is why I found the research results in the nalaxone trial so interesting.

The "monoamine theory" of why exercise helps treat depression essentially proposes that -

A) Depression is associated with low levels of serotonin, dopamine and/or norepinephrine.
B) Exercise has been shown to increase levels of all three of these monoamines
C) Therefore, exercise should help treat depression

Research has consistently demonstrated that exercise has reliable and beneficial effects on levels of serotonin, dopamine and norepinephrine (hereafter - 5-HT, DA and NE respectively).

Dopamine, which is responsible for a large part of your motivation (towards important goals such as food or sex) and pleasure, has been strongly implicated in depression. This is particularly the case for depression which is characterized by a lack of motivation and an inability to feel pleasure (anhedonia). In mice tests, rodents subjected to periods of forced exercise show significantly higher levels of dopamine in their brains.

Parkinson's disease is caused by a loss of dopaminergic neurons in the part of the brain responsible for movement. Remember, DA is not just involved in psychological motivation towards a particular goal, but also physical movement towards something also. Research into Parkinson's disease also appears to indicate that physical activity provides a degree of protection for dopaminergic neurons that would otherwise be vulnerable to toxicity induced damage.

NE (also known as noradrenaline) is also vital for physiological arousal and motivation towards important goals. However, chronic stress and depression are often associated with levels of NE that are far too high. This is particularly the case for scenarios where anxiety is present. Through a complex series of reactions in your brain, exercise appears to suppress NE levels in key areas of the brain. The result is that exercise appears to provide a degree of protection against chronic stress by reducing levels of NE.

There is also a related theory regarding NE which says that anxiety disorders are associated with a fight-or-flight response that is followed by neither fight nor flight. For example, if you are anxious about something, your body is flooded with stress hormones and neurotransmitters, with NE being central to the physical and psychological reaction. The purpose of this is to give you the energy or power to either fight the source of the threat or run away. If you do neither of these things, it is believed that NE just continues to float around your system, keeping you unnecessarily aroused. Therefore, by going out for a run, you are acting in sympathy with your physiology, burning off the excess stress hormones.

5-HT is the neurotransmitter most famously associated with depression. Selective serotonin re-uptake inhibitors (SSRIs) such as Prozac (fluoxetine) or Zoloft (sertraline) work by blocking the re-uptake of serotonin, leading to increased levels in the synapse (the space between neurons - or the space between axons and dendrites, to be specific). Exercise has consistently been shown to increase levels of serotonin in key areas of the brain such as the hippocampus (problems with the hippocampus is strongly implicated in depression).

However the problem with serotonin is that it is not a simple case of "more = better" throughout the brain. In fact, there is considerable debate as to whether SSRI drugs work because they increase levels of serotonin. Some people believe that work by healing the hippocampus or decreasing inflammation. For example, there are a range of serotonin receptor sub-types with a wide range of effects. Some receptors are involved in mood, others involved in nausea (anti-emetic drugs work by modulating these particular receptors), whereas others are involved in sleep cycles. Therefore, you cannot simply say that increasing serotonin fixes all of your problems. However, importantly, exercise appears to work in all the right places in terms of healing depression.

Irrespective of exactly what neurotransmitter is most important for exercise-mediated recovery from depression, it is clear that there is a strong link. In their review of all the clinical literature, *Exercise Benefits Brain Function: The Monoamine Connection*, Tzu-Wei Lin and Yu-Min Kuo state *"An overwhelming majority of studies accredit that the monoamine systems mediate the exercise-induced enhancement of various brain functions."*

### C) The *"Brain Derived Neurotrophic Factor* (BDNF)" Theory
One of the leading theories as to how antidepressant drugs treat depression is that they increase levels of BDNF, which is a kind of "fertilizer" for the brain. BDNF is required for *neurogenesis*, which is where new brain cells (neurons) are created, leading to *plastic* changes in the brain. For example, neurogenesis in the hippocampus is believed to be one of the keys to recovering from depression. The hippocampi of depressed people tends to show atrophy (reduction in activity or even mass), which also tends to normalise as patients recover.

What do you think is the single most powerful thing you can do to increase levels of BDNF? Yes, you guessed it - physical exercise.

An example of how everything is interrelated can be found in the connection between BDNF and serotonin (5-HT). As you may recall, one of the ways that SSRI drugs appear to treat depression is by increasing levels of BDNF via increased levels of serotonin. So whether the benefits for depression come from exercise increasing serotonin which increases BDNF or whether exercise directly increases BDNF independent of serotonin, the effect itself appears to be clear.

By the way, if you are serious about increasing BDNF, after exercise, probably the most powerful ways of increasing levels is by supplementing with curcumin, a substance extracted from turmeric. Along with omega-3 fatty acids, turmeric is one of the most powerful supplements for mood and brain health available.

### D) The Sense of Accomplishment Theory
Prominent researcher Kelly Lambert released a paper on depression which proposed the idea that *effort-based rewards* were a key component of recovering from depression. Lambert proposed that one of the most effective means for treating depression was focusing on achieving goals through effort. While there may be debate whether this is related to increased dopamine (your brain releases dopamine

as a kind of reward when it thinks you are achieving important goals that may help your survival) or just feeling good through a sense of accomplishment, the effect seems clear. Getting out of bed or off the sofa and out achieving a hard-won goal is a fast and effective way to treat depression.

This is proposed as one of the reasons why exercise is an effective treatment for depression. Achieving goals through exercise appears to stimulate your brain's reward circuit, leading to increased feelings of pleasure.

And the bonus is that this also appears to be the reason why patients who recover from depression through exercise stay happier for longer than those who recovered via antidepressant drugs. In the case of medication, consciously or subconsciously, there is the sense that the pill did all the work. Whereas in the case of exercise, *you* did all the work. You controlled the situation and healed yourself. This sends a powerful message to your brain that you remain in control of your situation. Remember, in all the famous mouse tests, when you take away the animal's sense of control over its environment, depression and anxiety invariably result.

### D) The "Circuit-breaker for Rumination" Theory
One of the hallmarks of depression is endless rumination, where you are trapped inside your own head, mulling endlessly over how bad your life has become. Most of the time your life is nowhere near as bad as you think. Unfortunately the other hallmark of depression is overly negative filters, where you interpret everything as negative, despite how positive or neutral it may be.
   Experts believe that rumination is one of the most insidious aspects of depression and one of the main reasons why it can continue for a long time. People get into the habit of endlessly thinking negative thoughts. As Cognitive Behavioral Therapy shows us, if you think negative thoughts all day, it's only natural that you would be in a bad mood.
   Therefore, at the very least, exercise serves as a useful distraction. To give an example - it would be very hard to ruminate in the middle of a soccer match with your friends or playing a few sets of tennis.
   I think negative rumination is like being a record stuck in a groove or a train on tracks. Exercise can work to jolt you out of your funk and get you out of your stuck groove. I have experienced this myself, where I have days where I am at a loose end, without anything to do and I feel my mood slowly drift lower during the day for no apparent reason. After a while of thinking "wow I am in a bad mood today" I will then force myself to hit the gym or go for a jog. As if by miracle, when I get back and take a shower, I find myself in a better mood for the rest of the day. All it often takes is that first initial jolt, which exercise so effectively provides. One thing I will notice is that even if I think about the things that were getting me down while I am exercising, I suddenly seem to think about the same things in a much more optimistic and positive way. Or to put it another way, what originally felt like a hopeless or depressing situation can suddenly be seen with a little more space and clarity. Exercise seems to give people that space and a clearer perspective.

### E) The "Tolerance to Unpleasant Sensations" Theory
Exercise can sometimes be unpleasant, depending on how far you push yourself. "No pain, no gain" can be true, to some extent. However, unfortunately (or fortunately), depression is often associated with a poor level of tolerance for

unpleasant sensations. An everyday headache or stomach-ache can be unbearable for depressed people sometimes.

For example, many studies have shown that if you subject someone to a stimuli that slowly gets more intense, depressed patients will indicate that it has become "painful" with much less pressure than non-depressed patients. Imagine a sharp object pushing into your arm, where you can accurately measure the amount of pressure being applied. To put it simply, a depressed patient will indicate that it is painful at around, say, 5 units of pressure. Whereas a non-depressed patient will go to 7 units before they indicate that there is pain.

Remember, pain and depression are closely linked. This is the reason that fibromyalgia patients struggled for many years to get doctors to acknowledge their condition. Their doctors initially just believed it was a facet of depression manifesting as perceived physical pain.

So, by subjecting yourself to controlled doses of unpleasant sensations each time you exercise, you are training yourself to be able to handle more and more "pain". Remember, the key is control – you have decided to go and exercise, so you remain in control of the amount of discomfort. I always point out the famous mouse tests which show us that if you subject a mouse to pain which it has no control over, depression and anxiety will be the likely result.

Exercise, to put it another way, toughens you up.

So now that you have read about the main theories, I think you can guess what I am going to say regarding which one I believe is correct. Yep, all of them. I think there are clearly many factors at play – some more strongly than others in certain people – however there are clearly a multitude of factors behind the effectiveness of exercise for depression.

I am always uncomfortable pointing to a single neurotransmitter or a group of neurotransmitters as being the sole factor in any mood disorder. I think this type of thinking tends to oversimplify a situation. This is why there is such debate around depression being caused by a "chemical imbalance". There is no single test that will measure how much serotonin is floating around your system. Coupled with this is the fact that measuring levels of serotonin (or metabolites of serotonin) in your blood is a poor indicator of serotonin levels in the brain.

Another example of this is when scientists first noticed elevated endorphin levels in runners. There was much excitement around this discovery until it was pointed out that the particular type of endorphins measured (there are many sub-types of endorphins in your brain and body) don't cross the blood-brain barrier. Anything that cannot pass the blood-brain barrier will not be able to have any psychological effects. So clearly there is more at work than just serotonin or just endorphins.

Also, some of the theories regarding exercise and neurotransmitters is conflicting, which suggests that there is more to the picture than we currently understand. For example, one theory of why exercise helps depression is that it increases levels of norepinephrine. One of the earliest studies appeared to show increased levels of one of the by-products of norepinephrine in people who exercised. However, another theory as to how exercise helps anxiety says that exercise burns up the norepinephrine floating around your system, leading to lower levels, which allows serotonin to dominate and cause you to feel calm.

Similarly, there is a theory which says that exercise burns through cortisol (your primary stress hormone which works together with norepinephrine). Cortisol is well known as being toxic for the brain in large amounts or in chronic, long-term doses. Cortisol is often fingered as the culprit for hippocampal atrophy which is often seen with depressed patients. So, as with the other theories, I do believe that cortisol is part of the answer, but not the whole answer.

However, what I will say is that the concept of achievement and personal mastery is what sets exercise apart from medication. To put it another way, I am not particularly amazed that exercise could increase serotonin and therefore treat depression. But at the end of the day, you could just take a pill to achieve the same effect and with much less effort.

It is the ability of exercise to heal depression via your own effort that sets it apart from other treatments. That is the one that most excites me

## Putting it into Practice

So now you know that exercise is a powerful treatment for depression and some of the theories as to why this may be the case. The next natural question must surely be - *What is the best form of exercise for treating depression and how do I put this knowledge into practice?*

I have read many clinical studies and books with convincing research data supporting particular types of exercise as being the "best" for treating depression. Some indicate that intense cardiovascular exercise which is short and intense is the best. Others say that weight training is better. However, despite all the convincing research, it appears as if just about any form of physical movement can be helpful. For example, for many people, the most powerful "antidepressant" they ever used was good old fashioned walking! In fact, recently I read a story regarding a particular actor who suffered intense anxiety and depression all of his life. One of his doctors instructed him to head out for a walk each morning after he woke up. This particular actor expressed amazement at just how powerful this simple act was in healing his depression.

Herein lies the problem with many of the theories of why exercise heals depression. For example, a simple walk around a park in no way stimulates the production of endorphins, yet it appears to treat depression. Why should this be the case? This is one of the most convincing arguments supporting the theory that exercise gives people a sense of accomplishment.

For a depressed person, just getting out of bed, into your shoes and out on the street for a walk can take superhuman effort. Once someone smashes through that invisible barrier, there can be a huge sense of achievement.

So that is why my recommendation is a simple, one-size-fits-all approach.

*Do whatever you are interested in doing or find enjoyable. Otherwise, whatever you do will not be sustainable.*

If you hate jogging, why punish yourself with something you don't want to do? If you are depressed, it may take quite an effort to get out and do something you enjoy, let alone something you hate. If you try to force yourself to do something you hate, you may struggle to stay at it. This is only going to compound any self-esteem issues you may have.

To help you decided on an appropriate activity, let me give you some points to consider -
- Choose something simple to do. Don't pick something located far away or involves a complicated set-up. For many, that is the beauty of jogging - you just put on a pair of shoes and start putting one leg in front of the other in a vigorous fashion!
- A team sport combines two of the most powerful antidepressants known - exercise and social interaction. Joining or creating a team with your friends would be ideal.
- Avoid sports or activities with too much danger involved. If you think you are depressed now, try adding a broken leg into the mix.
- Another powerful combination activity is yoga, which combines peaceful meditation with endorphin-stimulating stretches. I have come out of intense yoga classes high as a kite with endorphins flying around my brain.
- While exercising, it is important that you don't allow yourself to ruminate, running your troubles over and over in your mind. Practice mindfulness while you exercise, focusing on all the sensations you may be experiencing. One of my favourite techniques is to focus on both the pleasure and pain in a neutral way. I like to say in my head "ah...there is a stimuli that I interpret as pleasure" or "ah...there is a stimuli that I interpret as pain".
- Try to think of activities which provide a compounding benefit, like team sports where you add socialisation to exercise to achieve a kind of synergy. Other examples could be -
  - Swimming in the ocean (exercise plus salt water plus cool and refreshing)
  - Exercising in the sun (exercise plus vitamin D benefits - try to get 20 minutes without sunscreen (sunscreen blocks out vitamin D as well as UVA + UVB))
  - Gardening (exercise plus effort-based rewards)
  - Spring cleaning the house (exercise plus effort-based rewards plus a cleaner living space - there is nothing more depressing than being depressed in a house that looks like a pig sty)
  - Weight training (exercise plus improved self-esteem via improved body image)
  - If you are a parent, playing sport with your children (exercise plus self-esteem benefits).

Based on the compelling research which is gradually accumulating in support of exercise therapy for depression, I am confident that it will gradually form a greater part of mainstream therapy as time goes on. Herein lies the opportunity for you to get ahead of the curve and take advantage of a therapeutic modality that has a range of benefits over and above your recovery from depression.

Antidepressant medication has become an easy target these days, with many blaming "*big pharma*" for pushing these drugs onto an unsuspecting public. However I believe that this is not a fair assessment. For the severely depressed, antidepressants (which usually means SSRIs nowadays) are proven to be effective beyond any doubt, for the great majority of patients. And while these drugs can have a range of unpleasant side-effects such as sexual dysfunction and emotional blunting, these side-effects have nothing on past drugs. If you go back twenty or thirty years to the time of tricyclic antidepressants and monoamine oxidase inhibitors, there was often a huge price to pay in terms of side-effects.

Despite the success of modern day antidepressants for treating severe depression or anxiety, for milder cases the cost-benefit (cost being side-effects in this case) does not usually stack up. You are exposing yourself to a range of unpleasant side-effects with the strong chance of seeing no therapeutic benefit in return.

This is where other treatments such as exercise therapy comes in. So whether you are currently depressed and looking for an effective treatment, or whether you would like to inoculate yourself against becoming depressed, the answer is clear – get moving!

# Chapter 5 – Optimize your brain with nootropic supplements

For a long time now I have felt that too much great research information is buried deep in PubMed (where scientists publish their studies and the results of clinical trials) and is written in hard to understand language for the non-scientists out there (i.e. – most of us!).

This is particularly the case regarding nootropics, which are substances that improve an aspect of brain function such as – speed of thought, memory, creativity or mood. For example, almost no-one outside of specialized circles has even heard of something like piracetam, to give just one example.

This is a shame because many people just accept cognitive decline as part of the aging process or as an unfortunate yet unavoidable side-effect of certain medications. If there is one thing I would like you to realise from reading this guide, it is that you do have means of reversing cognitive decline or low mood through powerful supplements.

## Omega 3 Fatty Acids

I have put omega 3 fatty acids at number one as I believe they are the single most important substance for a healthy brain. Unless you are living on a traditional Inuit diet, everybody should be taking omega 3 supplements. Off the top of my head I cannot think of another supplement which I believe to be compulsory for just about everybody.

Large parts of your brain are made of omega 3 Fatty Acids. Particularly the myelin, which covers your neurons and enables normally brain functioning. The disease multiple sclerosis involves the loss of functioning of the myelin so you can see how important this fatty sheath is for your nervous system. (I should point out here that omega 3 deficiency is not suspected as a primary cause of multiple sclerosis. At the time of writing this, the leading candidate for this is an inflammatory and autoimmune problem potentially mediated by Vitamin D. However we do not yet know for sure)

You may also have heard of omega 6 fatty acids, which you mostly get from consuming grains or meat from animals that were fed grains. Omega 6 is also important for you; however the modern diet has far too much omega 6 at the expense of omega 3. Why is this a problem? Omega 6 is pro-inflammatory. This means that your body uses Omega 6 to produce substances which cause inflammation to fight certain illness and injury. However if you consume too much omega 6 and not enough omega 3, inflammation can get out of hand. We are currently seeing an epidemic of inflammatory diseases in modern society such as – rheumatoid arthritis, multiple sclerosis (as I just mentioned), heart disease and cancer. Inflammation of the brain, along with chronic stress (which also exacerbates inflammation) is toxic for your brain.

Some scientists now believe that one of the causes of depression is chronic inflammation of the brain. Omega 3 supplements are also used successfully to treat those suffering from bipolar disease. It is believed that omega 3 helps normalise the dysfunctional nerve impulses in the brain associate with this condition. Some trials have also shown that omega 3 supplementation has been beneficial in slowing the onset of dementia in the elderly.

You should endeavour to decrease your consumption of omega 6 rich foods and increase your consumption of omega 3 foods (particularly fatty fish). Unfortunately, if you are consuming the standard western diet, it is unlikely that you will be able to normalise the omega 3 to 6 ratio with food alone. Therefore I strongly recommend adding omega 3 supplements to your regime.

I favour constantly mixing up my source of omega 3, as each source has different ratios of DHA (Docosahexaenoic acid) & EPA (Eicosapentaenoic acid) which are the two fatty acids which make up most sources of Omega 3. Here are some different sources –

- General Fish Oil
- Krill Oil
- Cod Liver Oil (also contains Vitamin D and Vitamin A)
- Seafood (particularly fatty fish such as salmon & sardines)
- Grass fed beef

As a final quick warning, make sure you go easy on any fish known to contain traces of mercury. This usually means predatory fish at the top of the food chain such as shark, swordfish or tuna

## Acetyl L-Carnitine (ALCAR)

ALCAR, which is the acetylated form of the amino acid l-carnitine, is an important substance for the brain which improves memory and concentration via its beneficial action on the neurotransmitter acetylcholine. Acetylcholine is one of the major neurotransmitters in the brain responsible for maintaining focused attention and clear thinking. Problems with acetylcholine can result in neurological conditions such as Alzheimer's. Indeed, many of the major treatments for Alzheimer's focus on normalising levels of acetylcholine.

Alzheimer's is not the only neurological disease where ALCAR has shown promise. Due to beneficial effects on your brain's dopamine system, ALCAR has also been investigated as an adjunct treatment for Parkinson's disease. However, you don't have to be suffering from Parkinson's to gain benefit from ALCAR, which provides mood and memory benefits to everyone via the powerful effects on your dopaminergic system.

ALCAR has also been shown to act as a powerful antioxidant in the brain, repairing various forms of environmental and age-related damage. Indeed, this damage-repairing aspect of ALCAR has seen it being investigated as a way to accelerate the healing process after a major stroke.

ALCAR is also well known as one of the best agents for improving mitochondrial function, alongside other important substances such as co-enzyme Q10. Your mitochondria is your individual cells' powerhouse, producing energy throughout the brain and body at a cellular level. As you can imagine, it is therefore extremely important that your mitochondrial system is functioning optimally.

Due to either the mitochondrial or the dopaminergic effects, ALCAR has also demonstrated good effectiveness at treating some of the pain and cognitive dysfunction associated with fibromyalgia, an incurable neuropathic pain condition which affects millions of people around the world.

Alpha Lipoic Acid (ALA)

It is impossible to explain the benefits of alpha lipoic acid (ALA) for the brain without first explaining exactly what glutathione is. Glutathione is like the body's 'master antioxidant', repairing damage and increasing the effectiveness of other antioxidants you consume, such as vitamin C and vitamin E. If Glutathione was able to be taken effectively as a supplement it would be on this list. Unfortunately, consuming Glutathione does not increase levels in your body by any measurable amount.

Fortunately there are other supplements which have been shown to dramatically increase levels of glutathione, of which ALA is one of the main examples. As glutathione is vital for keeping your brain young and healthy, it is hardly surprising that ALA supplementation has shown the ability to slow down and even reverse the cognitive dysfunction associated with old age.

This brain-repairing characteristic of ALA is the reason why it is also being studied to treat some of the symptoms of serious neurological conditions such as Alzheimer's and MS. ALA appears to repair damage to cell walls, providing further clues as to why this supplement is getting so much attention from researchers.

As inflammation is one of the prime suspects in chronic brain damage and premature aging, it is also not surprising that ALA has been shown to exert anti-inflammatory effects on the brain also.

Phosphatidylserine (PS)

PS makes up a large part of the membrane around your brain's cells and is consequently vital for smooth communication between cells.
Supplementation has been shown to improve not only concentration and memory in healthy subjects, but also improved mood in subjects suffering from depression.

One of the most exciting applications of PS therapy is in the treatment of ADD and ADHD. The positive effects of PS supplementation on concentration is powerful evidence for the beneficial effects on the human brain.

Another study showed that PS supplementation reduced levels of cortisol in the brain. Chronically elevated cortisol (usually from stress, mood disorders or excessive exercise) is toxic to the brain. For example, this has been shown to measurably decrease the size of the human hippocampus - a part of the brain vital for memory and mood. Substances such as PS, which can reduce cortisol levels in the brain, are therefore extremely important for avoiding damage caused by chronic stress.

N-Acetylcysteine (NAC)

Remember that wonderful glutathione I mentioned before? NAC is probably the most powerful known agent for increasing levels of glutathione.

You have probably heard of those people who die of liver failure after taking an overdose of acetaminophen (paracetamol). The reason why overdosing on this common painkiller can cause liver failure is that it is a toxic substance which the liver uses glutathione to detoxify. In normal doses this doesn't create any problems, however in overdose, your liver simply runs out of glutathione and liver failure often follows. Guess what is often given to these emergency room patients? Yes – NAC.

The beauty of NAC is that the beneficial effects are not just limited to the brain. Your whole body benefits – particularly your liver, as you could imagine, considering the example I just gave.

Due to the dramatic effects on glutathione, NAC is a powerful agent for preventing and repairing damage to the brain from toxins or the aging process.
NAC has been shown to be effective at reducing the symptoms of obsessive compulsive disorder (OCD). It does this by reducing levels of certain neurotransmitters which put the brain of an OCD sufferer into overdrive. For this same reason, NAC has shown promise also as an effective treatment for schizophrenia and bi-polar disorder.

For a fantastic guide dedicated to this amazing substance, I highly recommend you check out James Lee's book on NAC.

## Choline, Alpha GPC & Citicoline (CDP Choline)

Choline is a vital nutrient used extensively throughout the brain. Like PS, it makes up part of cell membranes. Also, as with omega 3 and PS, you can think of choline as a substance the brain uses to make itself and repair itself.

As you would imagine from the name, supplementary choline is also used by the brain to produce acetylcholine, which, as you saw previously, is vital for memory and other cognitive functions. Not only this, choline is also used to produce trimethylglycine (TMG) and S-Adenosylmethionine (SAM-e), two substances which are strongly implicated in positive mood. SAM-e is itself available as a mood-boosting supplement, however Choline supplementation may be a cheaper way of boosting levels of SAM-e in the brain. I should also point out that trimethylglycine itself is also a powerful and cost effective mood booster.

The major source of choline in the diet is one of my favourite super-foods – the humble egg. If you consume plenty of eggs, you probably do not need to supplement additional choline, however several studies have shown that the average westerner is deficient in choline. Not only this, but a study showed that the greater this deficiency of choline was, the more anxious a person was likely to be.

Another important indicator of how choline is used to build your brain, a very interesting study showed a positive relationship between a mother's consumption of choline and higher IQ in their children.

Choline has also been shown to reduce damage to the brain associated with alcoholism. Indeed, some people recommend a large meal of eggs when you have a hangover due to the high choline content.

There are three main ways you can deliver forms of choline to your brain or to boost levels – straight choline supplements, alpha GPC or CDP choline (also known as citicoline). Each of these has different studies demonstrating potential in different areas. Personally I am more favourable towards citicoline and alpha GPC because often it is not a shortage of choline which is to blame, but some other step in the process.

CDP-choline is precursor for the production of phosphatidylcholine and is one step further along the chain from straight choline. Put another way, your brain makes CDP-choline out of choline before it is then made into phosphatidylcholine. CDP-choline has been shown to be beneficial for a range of conditions including ADHD and Alzheimer's and also assist in the recovery from a stroke. CDP-choline is neuro-protective, via positive effects on levels of glutathione, phosphatidylcholine and by reducing oxidative stress and inflammation in the brain. CDP-choline has also been shown to improve cognition (thinking ability) in the brain by improving glucose metabolism (glucose is your brain's primary source of fuel).

Alpha GPC is essentially a by-product of the metabolic process which creates phosphatidylcholine. Despite coming in at a different stage in the process, alpha GPC essentially does the same thing as CDP-choline and has been studied for the same conditions.

Despite the fact that CDP-choline and alpha GPC essentially do very similar things, users often report dramatically different results depending on which one they use. I therefore recommend you experiment before deciding which one works best for you.

Most of the research around CDP-choline and alpha GPC is focused around Alzheimer's and Parkinson's disease. This is due to the strong interrelation between acetylcholine (Alzheimer's) and dopamine (Parkinson's). Indeed, in an interesting trial, adding CDP-choline to L-DOPA (a standard Parkinson's treatment), dramatically increased the effectiveness of the therapy.

Inositol

Inositol is a type of sugar which forms a key component of brain lipids (fatty parts of your brain). You will remember from previous sections that some of the other vital components of your brain cell membranes are omega 3 and phosphatidylserine.

Inositol has been extensively studied for its beneficial effects on various aspects of mood. Due to this property, inositol has been used as a novel antidepressant and as a treatment for OCD, panic disorder and bi-polar. The reason for inositol's beneficial effects on mood appear to be via its important role in healthy neurotransmission. As you may know, faulty neurotransmitter activity which reduces levels of serotonin, dopamine and norepinephrine is theorized to be behind many mood disorders.

Inositol appears to have a synergistic effect with choline. Meaning, by combining choline with inositol, there appears to be more benefit than with either on its own. This is why many supplements are a combination of choline + inositol.

Piracetam

Of all the supplements mentioned in this guide, perhaps the most powerful is piracetam, which is a type of substance called a *racetam*. Racetams are considered to be the 'next big thing' in the field of nootropics due to the powerful effects they can have on the brain. In fact, piracetam can have effects closer to a drug than a typical dietary supplement.

While racetams have positive effects in all kinds of different areas of the brain, due to how new this class of supplements are, scientists are still trying to work out exactly how racetams work in some cases. Like many of the other supplements on this list, racetams have positive effects on acetylcholine, improving memory and cognition in most cases.

Piracetam also appears to have a positive effect on NMDA glutamate receptors, which are central to learning and memory. This beneficial effect is further increased due to the fact that piracetam increases oxygen consumption in the brain, improving brain health and function.

This incredible substance improves an amazing range of conditions including – Alzheimer's, stroke, childhood autism and depression. However its main use is still as the 'poster child' for nootropics, used by students 'in the know' to improve cognition and memory, leading to better test scores.

Many ADHD sufferers who have been on stimulants such as Ritalin or Adderall long term, use piracetam to repair some of the damage done to their brains from stimulant use. Using stimulants is like driving a car at full throttle, increasing wear and tear. Piracetam appears to offset this wear and tear to a certain extent.

One drawback of Piracetam is that it only seems to have positive effects for some people. Many people claim they saw no positive effects or even some negative effects. You will need to see whether it works for you or not

Vitamin D

Vitamin D is not really a vitamin; it is a fat soluble steroid hormone that is mostly obtained from sun exposure and through foods which contain vitamin D, such as eggs or organ meats. When your skin is exposed to the sun, it triggers a reaction which creates vitamin D in the body – you don't actually 'absorb' vitamin D from the sun itself.

Studies consistently show that the general population in the west is often deficient in Vitamin D. This is due to the various factors such as –

- To be 'sun smart' and reduce our risk of skin cancer, many people now avoid sun exposure. Surprisingly, a large percentage of the population in sunny locations such as Florida are even vitamin D deficient.
- Humans evolved to eat organ meats (such as liver and kidney) of animals they killed, whereas now, most meat eaters only consume muscle meat. Organ meats are naturally high in dietary vitamin D

Darker skinned people have more trouble in obtaining enough Vitamin D from the sun and therefore need to consume more in their diet. From an evolutionary perspective this is quite interesting as people closer to the equator (where it is sunniest) tend to have darker skin than people from the far north and the far south. It appears as if evolution has created a natural balancing mechanism for vitamin D absorption. In modern times this has been upset by our propensity to now migrate over large latitudinal distances.

Due to the vital role played by Vitamin D in the brain, scientists now believe that a lack of vitamin D may be one of the causes of MS. This was discovered when researchers began to notice that the closer people live to the poles (i.e. – in cold countries with less sunshine), the greater the prevalence of MS. We are a long way from conclusively proving the link between vitamin D and MS, however it is an extremely promising line of investigation nonetheless.

In terms of effects, vitamin D is involved in producing various neurotrophins in the brain. These are substances involved in creating and growing new brain cells. For example, certain neurotrophins are recognised as the brain's version of 'fertilizer', helping individual neurons to grow healthily.

As with many of the supplements in this guide, vitamin D acts as a powerful anti-inflammatory, cooling down inflammation in the brain.

Vitamin D has become hot property lately in research circles, being implicated in conditions as varied as autism, Alzheimer's and Parkinson's disease

The biggest mistake people make when supplementing vitamin D is forgetting to add vitamin K. It has long been known that vitamin D increases your absorption of calcium – hence the fact that most supplements for osteoporosis contain both calcium and vitamin D. However researchers recently discovered that vitamin K is what directs your body to lay down the dietary calcium in your bones. Without vitamin K, if you take large amounts of vitamin D, there is a possibility that your body could lay down the calcium in the worst possible place – your arteries.  Therefore, always make sure you take vitamin K with your vitamin D supplements.

I recommend mixing up your sources of dietary Vitamin D, including –

- Straight vitamin D + vitamin K supplements
- Cod liver oil Supplements (don't take too much of this though as it has high levels of Vitamin A which can be toxic in overdose)
- Foods such as eggs & liver

The beauty of sun exposure (apart from being cost free) is that your body has a mechanism for turning off vitamin D production when you have enough.  Dietary vitamin D does not have this benefit and there is controversy over whether high doses of dietary Vitamin D are beneficial or toxic.  Just limit your exposure to 20-30 minutes a day, without sunscreen, and you will not be increasing your chances developing skin cancer.

## B-Group Vitamins

When we talk about B-group vitamins, we are talking about a whole host of different vitamins which get lumped together and referred to as "B-group vitamins". As a group, they are just about the most important class of vitamins for the brain, which is why any supplement you buy for reducing stress levels usually contains B-group vitamins.

As a group, they are water soluble, so your body doesn't retain them in its fat stores. You therefore need to consume them on a regular basis as your body cannot 'retain' any excess you consume, as it does with fat-soluble vitamins like vitamin E.

The only time I would recommend you to buy the B-vitamins separately is if you have a particular condition that needs high doses of one of the B-vitamins, or if you have a genetic issue which requires a different form of one of the B-vitamins. For example, some people cannot utilize folic acid and therefore need to supplement with L-methylfolate, which is further down the metabolic chain. Therefore, the best way to cover all bases is by taking a Multi-B or Mega B each day. One of these tablets will usually have all of the B-group vitamins in just the right doses to prevent deficiency.

To break it down further, some of the key members of this group include –

**Thiamine (B1)** - Your brain needs thiamine for oxidative metabolism and for producing acetylcholine in the brain. Deficiency in thiamine can cause devastating brain diseases such as Beriberi and Wernicke-Korsakoff syndrome.

**Riboflavin (B2)** – Riboflavin is a vital component of Glutathione synthesis, so if you have gone to the trouble of taking supplements to increase glutathione and you are deficient in riboflavin, you will be wasting your time.

**Niacin (B3)** - A recent study showed that niacin helped the brain to rewire itself after a stroke and that niacin protects against Alzheimer's and other age-related brain disorders. Deficiency in niacin leads to a serious disease called Pellagra.
Pantothenic Acid (B5) - Many people take Pantothenic Acid to assist in memory and concentration due to its vital importance for synthesizing acetylcholine.

**Pyridoxine (B6)** - Pyridoxine is vital for the production of neurotransmitters such as serotonin, dopamine and noradrenaline. Consequently, a lack of pyroxidine in the diet has been strongly implicated in depression and anxiety.

**Biotin (B7)** - Biotin is vital for the metabolism of fatty acids in the brain and for the proper functioning of neurons. Biotin deficiency can lead to a host of neurological conditions such as seizures.

**Folic Acid (B9)** - Folic Acid is most famous as a supplement that expecting mothers can take to prevent neural tube defects in their baby. However it is also vital for the brain. Particularly for the way the brain produces and uses serotonin and noradrenaline. Folic Acid is so important for serotonin production that it is sometime prescribed alongside antidepressants to increase their effectiveness. As previously mentioned, some people have problems metabolising dietary folate correctly and should therefore take a separate supplement on top of their Multi B, called L-methylfolate.

**Cobalamin (B12)** - Studies have shown that people with B12 deficiency perform poorly on cognitive tests, with higher consumption linked to lower levels of Alzheimer's disease. A deficiency of B12 is linked to lethargy, lack of motivation and sleeping problems. B12 is difficult to absorb from food (it has what is called low bioavailability). So if you are deficient, you need to either get B12 injections or use sublingual tablets (you put under your tongue to absorb into the bloodstream, not via your stomach).

## Noopept

One of the newer and perhaps more obscure nootropics is Noopept, which is a proprietary peptide originating out of Russia. It shares a molecular similarity with the racetams but with significantly greater potency. One of the reasons for this is that Noopept has comparatively favorable blood-brain barrier crossing abilities. The blood-brain barrier is a kind of membrane the brain utilizes as a protective mechanism. Many molecules cannot pass through and are therefore rendered inactive. For example, this is one of the reasons why a depressed person can't just take serotonin as a supplement - serotonin is not able to cross this barrier. The closest you can get is to take serotonin's direct precursor, 5-htp, which can indeed cross the blood-brain barrier to an extent.

As Noopept is related to the racetams, unsurprisingly it has similar neuro-protective effects on the brain. The memory-boosting effects in particular have been extensively verified in animal testing.

One of the holy grails of nootropics is to isolate substances which stimulate the production or expression of NGF (Nerve growth factor) or BDNF (Brain-derived neurotrophic factor), which act as a kind of 'fertilizer' for the brain. Noopept has been shown to indeed possess this characteristic, with serum levels of these important growth factors increasing after administration with Noopept.

The guinea pigs for Noopept have been the Russians, who take it as a nootropic to improve learning ability and memory. Studies have also shown that Noopept has the ability to repair certain aspects of brain dysfunction after major injury such as a stroke.

As with many other nootropics, Noopept also appears to have beneficial effects on mood. Subjects administered Noopept reported reduced anxiety, improved sleep and less mood swings. I should note however that I am unable to verify whether these factors were correctly placebo-controlled. As you could imagine, if you start taking a powerful cognitive enhancer, it would not be unthinkable for mood to improve as a secondary effect.

One thing I should point out is that, due to the fact that this is such a powerful nootropic, if you decided to try it, I recommend that you start out at a low, conservative dose. I have read reports of strange psychedelic-like effects for those who have pushed the dose too hard at the beginning. Also I recommend that you take regular breaks from Noopept (even if it is working well) as you will slowly build a tolerance to its effects. A short 1-2 week break should be sufficient to reset your tolerance.

One side-effect to look for is a slight increase in aggression. I suspect that Noopept has dopamine-boosting effects which could account for this. Substances which increase dopamine at the expense of serotonin and prolactin, can sometimes increase aggression. If you find yourself getting more aggressive or irritable than usual, stop Noopept immediately and look elsewhere for your nootropic stack.

I have surveyed some of the various nootropics-focused discussion boards and have found fairly consistent reporting of effects including –

- *Improved measures of perception including better visual acuity and better olfactory (smelling) faculties*
- *Dramatically improved memory*
- *Improved social skills and reduced social anxiety*
- *Potent mood-boosting*
- *Improved creativity and appreciation for the creative arts*

Sulbutiamine

As you will recall from the section on B-group vitamins, thiamine (B1) is an important vitamin for a healthy brain. Sulbutiamine is a synthetic derivative of thiamine which has been modified to enable it to cross the blood-brain barrier more easily.
In terms of effects on the brain, as well as the traditional nootropic effects such as improved memory and less social anxiety, Sulbutiamine also shows promise as a treatment for chronic fatigue syndrome (CFS), asthenia and erectile dysfunction.

However, out of these, it is the debilitating fatigue inducing condition asthenia where Sulbutiamine has shown the most promise. For example, the first trial for CFS appeared to show no statistically significant benefit over placebo.

As with most other nootropics, Sulbutiamine appears to improve memory function via the cholinergic, dopaminergic and glutaminergic pathways. Interestingly, a recent trial showed promise in adding Sulbutiamine to standard Alzheimer's drugs to improve various memory-related measures of that disorder. If you have Alzheimer's, please do not just commence Sulbutiamine therapy without involvement from your doctor. Alzheimer's is related to problems with acetylcholine (which Sulbutiamine influences), so you should never start tweaking your therapeutic regime without your doctor's agreement.

Sulbutiamine also improves various measures of social anxiety, indicating a potential adjunct treatment for those suffering from anxiety disorders or depression. A recent trial of patients with major depression seemed to show that Sulbutiamine administered for 4 weeks improved various aspect of social inhibition which is typical of this disorder. I should point out that this effect was observed independent of any antidepressant effect as Sulbutiamine did not confer any mood-boosting benefit to these subjects.

As with the other nootropics, I recommend you to start your dosage low, around 200mg per day. You can then increase as required or decrease if you start to experience intolerable side-effects. That said, Sulbutiamine appears to have no major side-effects, which is consistent with the fact that it is just a derivative of B1.

## Theanine

Theanine (sometimes referred to as "L-Theanine" is the amino acid found in tea (Camellia Sinensis) which is reportedly responsible for tea's mood-boosting effects. Since being isolated by Japanese researchers, theanine has gone on to become a popular nootropic and mood-booster around the world.

As theanine easily crosses the blood-brain barrier, it has various cognitive and psychoactive effects, including its ability to sooth stress, improve aspects of cognition and reduce fatigue. Theanine is perhaps most famously known for its ability to induce alpha waves in the brain, which are associated with feelings of relaxed alertness.

Despite the fact that theanine is related to glutamate (the brain's most prominent excitatory neurotransmitter), it's effects do not seem to come from interacting with glutamate receptors themselves. This reminds me a lot of the drug pregabalin (Lyrica) which is structurally related to the main inhibitory neurotransmitter GABA, but doesn't appear to agonize or antagonize the GABA receptors. Interestingly, one of the main effects of theanine in the brain is to increase levels of GABA, which would certainly account for the relaxation-inducing properties.

Another strange and interesting property of theanine is that it appears to increase levels of dopamine. This is interesting for the simple fact that dopaminergic agents usually cause excitation rather than relaxation. However this would certainly account for the reported improvements in concentration and focus. In terms of serotonin, the data is less clear. I had always assumed that theanine must work primarily via serotonin, however this doesn't seem to necessarily be the case.

As with most effective nootropics, animal studies have shown the theanine appears to have good neuro-protective effects, suggesting potential for repairing certain types of brain damage or aging.

A study on subjects with ADHD showed improvements in anxiety and sleep quality, perhaps helping to offset some of the adverse effects of stimulant medications used to treat this disorder.

While I support the use of theanine as a nootropic, I can't help but think that it would be a better course of action to obtain it from drinking tea (particularly green tea). This is for several reasons. Firstly, theanine has been consumed in this fashion for centuries throughout Asia, so the safety aspect is well established. Secondly, theanine works synergistically with caffeine, which means that the natural caffeine and theanine contained in tea should work together to increase the beneficial effects. Thirdly, green tea itself has many nootropic effects due to its action as a powerful antioxidant. Green tea contains the important chemical EGCG which has been shown to stimulate the production of neuronal cells via neurogenesis. This is particularly prominent in the hippocampus, the part of the brain associated with mood and memory.

## Huperzine A

Huperzine A is natural alkaloid compound, extracted from certain plants, which acts, among other things, as an acetylcholinesterase inhibitor. As you may recall, acetylcholinesterase inhibitors are a class of drug used to treat Alzheimer's disease. It is therefore unsurprising that a synthetic form of Huperzine A is currently being developed as a treatment for this devastating brain disease.

In recent times, Huperzine A has, despite being relatively unknown, started to become more popular as a nootropic supplement for memory support. For this use it has some good initial trial data to back it up as a memory-enhancer.

Huperzine A's ability to treat Alzheimer's does not come from only its action as a acetylcholinesterase inhibitor. Importantly, it also acts as an NMDA receptor antagonist - a relatively rare property for a plant-based extract. NMDA receptor antagonists act as nootropics by reducing levels of glutamate related excitatotoxicity. Think of this in terms of a brain stuck in high-gear leading to increased levels of wear and tear. Significantly, Huperzine A also increases levels of nerve growth factor, providing a further boost to your brain's rebuilding efforts.

However here is a key point worth expanding on - As with most nootropics, one man's medicine can be another's poison. Huperzine A's ability to act as an NMDA antagonist is only helpful if you have an overactive glutaminergic system. Remember, many nootropics do the exact opposite - they increase glutaminergic activity to 'turbo-charge' your brain, with learning being extensively modulated by glutamate.

Two disorders characterised by too much glutamate, which would possibly benefit from Huperzine A are Alzheimer's and Fibromyalgia. In fact, regarding Fibromyalgia, a recent paper recommended the use of two substances together - pregabalin (Lyrica) to reduce glutamate, and another Alzheimer's drug, memantine, to act as an NMDA antagonist.

One warning I should point out is that NMDA antagonists can sometimes cause issues for those with either diagnosed schizophrenia or a history of this condition in their family. If you have even the slightest doubt, I recommend you to avoid Huperzine A. However for all other people, this supplement appears to be relatively well-tolerated with minimal side-effects.

Curcumin

In the world of natural health, curcumin is fast becoming the new superstar - and for good reason. In terms of overall brain and body health, curcumin is near the top of my list for almost compulsory supplements (alongside Omega 3 of course!). Curcumin is the bioactive compound extracted from turmeric - yes the same turmeric you have in your curry! It therefore comes as no surprise that turmeric has a long history of use in India's traditional Ayurvedic system.

Curcumin has been studied for a huge range of conditions from arthritis to cancer, however in my opinion it is the effects of curcumin on the brain that warrant the most excitement.

Also, it is worth pointing out that curcumin is not just another 'woo woo' herb that only naturopaths recommend. There are currently a range of clinical trials under way studying curcumin for conditions such as depression or inflammatory disorders.

So why is curcumin such a powerful brain tonic? Well, there are several reasons however first and foremost curcumin is one of nature's most powerful anti-inflammatory substances. More and more, inflammation is now being implicated in a range of disorders emanating from the brain and nervous system. For example, a recent hypothesis has emerged from some scientists proposing that clinical depression is primarily and inflammatory problem. This is not new either. It has long been known that one of the strange secondary effects of SSRI antidepressants is that they also appear to act as anti-inflammatories.

I strongly believe that one of the number one brain destroyers over time is uncontrolled inflammation. One of the main reasons for this is the modern day shift in our diet from being heavy on Omega 3 fatty acids (anti-inflammatory) to Omega 6 fatty acids (pro-inflammatory). This is mainly due to our shift to grains (wheat etc) both in terms of what we eat but also what our meat eats - Meaning, livestock are now mostly fed grain instead of grass.

I should point out that it would be pointless to start taking curcumin to reduce inflammation if you maintain a highly pro-inflammatory diet. I read a great analogy for this recently - This would be like starting more fires at the same time you are calling the fire department (curcumin) to come and assist! In terms of simplicity, I highly recommend you investigate paleo-type diets which tend to be anti-inflammatory.

A good indication for the esteem in which curcumin is now held, it is currently being studied as an adjunct Alzheimer's treatment. As you know from the other nootropics in this book, drugs and supplements which treat Alzheimer's are often powerful nootropic agents. Curcumin appears to help with Alzheimer's symptoms by reducing inflammatory damage and reducing the formation of beta-amyloid plaque.

Curcumin is also a powerful mood-booster via its reduction of inflammation and its action as a MAOI (monoamine oxidase inhibitor). MAOIs inhibit the breakdown of serotonin, dopamine and norepinephrine in the brain, leading to improved mood.

One of the main reasons I recommend curcumin as a nootropic is its ability to increase levels of BDNF, which, as you may recall, is a kind of fertilizer for the brain. Apart from cardiovascular exercise, there are not many ways you can modulate BDNF, however curcumin is one.

One point I should make is that you need to buy curcumin which has added ingredients to make it more bioactive. Curcumin on its own has low bioavailability, which means that you need to take huge amounts to have any effect. Fortunately these new additives (such as piperine) effectively increase the amount of curcumin absorbed.

## Rhodiola Rosea

Chronic stress is often cited as the prime culprit for most cases of premature brain aging or non-trauma based injury to the brain. Put simply, chronic stress is terrible for your brain. I am not talking about acute stress, such as when you need to take an exam or make a presentation in front of a large group of people. Chronic stress is unending, day in day out, low level stress which put enormous stress on your brain and body.

One of the reasons why chronic stress is worse for your brain than acute stress is the toxic effects of cortisol. Cortisol is a glucocorticoid stress hormone secreted in response to stressful events. Cortisol is a vital hormone and there is nothing bad about it per se. The problem occurs when stress becomes chronic and cortisol levels remain constantly elevated.

Probably the most widely studied effect of elevated cortisol on the brain is reduced hippocampus function. Chronically elevated cortisol has clearly been shown to impact your hippocampus's ability to lay down new memories in an optimal fashion. One of the best supplements for neutralizing the effects of cortisol on the brain is the Arctic shrub Rhodiola Rosea, which has been used traditionally in Russia and Scandinavian countries for relieving stress and nervous disorders. And this is not just the realm of unproven traditional medicine - the ability of Rhodiola to reduce cortisol levels and normalize sensitivity of cortisol receptors has been proven in placebo-controlled trials.

The stress-reducing abilities of Rhodiola are mainly due to its ability to act as a powerful MAOI (monoamine oxidase inhibitor), thereby increasing levels of serotonin, dopamine and norepinephrine.

Rhodiola is now my first choice when recommending a natural antidepressant. The reason I recommend this ahead of St. John's Wort is that St. John's Wort can cause problematic interactions with other medications due to the fact that it changes the way your liver metabolizes certain drugs.

As with most nootropics or natural antidepressants, I recommend you to start on a low dose and gradually work up if you don't suffer any adverse effects. The best indication that you may be pushing things too hard will be if you start to feel anxious. If this happens, drop back down a dose and see how that works.

Also I should point out that in the area of monoamines, everybody is different. Some people may have too little serotonin, others too little dopamine. As Rhodiola is a broad spectrum MAOI, if your problem is specific to serotonin, you may become anxious or agitated, irrespective of dose. If this happens, move on to something else.

Bacopa Monnieri

Bacopa Monnieri is a nootropic herb with a long history in Indian Ayurvedic medicine, where it is known as Brahmi. In recent years it has gone from an obscure Ayurvedic herb to a staple of smart nootropic stacks.

Recently Bacopa Monnieri has demonstrated solid effects on the brain through multiple clinical trials. These trials appear to indicate potential for Bacopa Monnieri to improve various aspects of memory and cognition. One area of particular promise is using Bacopa Monnieri to reverse age-related cognitive decline in the elderly.

So how does it work? Well, this is where it gets a little complicated as Bacopa Monnieri appears to have a few different mechanisms of action. However each of these mechanisms fall broadly into the category of "antioxidants". Firstly, Bacopa Monnieri not only increases levels of our old friend glutathione, but also of related defenders against oxidative damage - superoxide dismutase and catalase. It appears as if some of the polyphenols in Bacopa Monnieri are responsible for its powerful antioxidant activity.

As with so many of the nootropics in this book, the 'canary in the coalmine' in terms of assessing whether Bacopa Monnieri is effective appears to be testing it on Alzheimer's patients. Whilst there have been no major trials on humans, in rodent trials, Bacopa Monnieri reduced levels of beta amyloid plaque which characterizes this disease.

One thing I should point out is that among nootropic aficionados, Bacopa Monnieri is known for its wide range of effects, depending on the person. For some people it gives them energy, for others it makes them sleepy. Whilst some people have seen no benefit whatsoever, among those who have benefited, an improvement in memory and cognition definitely appears to be a common theme.

Another regular comment I hear is that the effects differ between brands. As each brand can have different sources for the raw herbs or different extraction techniques, this is to be expected. So again, you may need to experiment with brand and dose to find your particular 'sweet spot'.

Other Options and Potential Future Inclusions

Due to the fact that just about anything you ingest has effects on the brain, the potential number of supplements I could include in this book is huge. I have therefore stuck to those that I consider to be powerful, effective, safe and with good research and experiential backing.

In case you wish to create a nootropic stack that includes certain supplements not included in this book, here is a list of some potential candidates which could warrant further investigation –

**Other racetams** – Piracetam is not the only option. There is also – oxiracetam, aniracetam and pramiracetam. Each seems to have a slightly different effect so if one doesn't work for you, it may be worth trying another racetam

**Gingko Biloba** – Mild MAOI and improves blood flow in the brain (possibly by acting as a mild blood thinner)

**Co-enzyme Q10** – Improves mitochondrial function

**Magnesium** – Reduces stress via neuromuscular relaxation.

**Zinc** – A vital co-factor for various brain processes

**Ashwagandha** – A powerful relaxation-inducing Indian herb

**Picamilon** – A powerful stress-reducing supplement – acts on GABA receptors in a similar fashion to benzodiazepine drugs such as Valium.

# Chapter 6 – Brain boosting games and activities

The human brain is not dissimilar to the muscles on and in your body. Just like muscles, the brain grows with use and shrinks with disuse.

One of the pioneers of neuroplasticity was Canadian psychologist Donald Hebb, who proposed the mechanism which underlies current day neuroplasticity. In essence, the theory can be boiled down to the simple statement that – repeating the same activity over and over will strengthen the connections in the brain related to that activity.

It is this theory which has led to the modern day concept of the 'brain gym', where you do certain mental activities repeatedly to 'grow' your brain in certain ways.

This concept has becoming increasingly popular in recent years as research continues to show that staying mentally active in old age is the best way to ward off dementia related diseases such as Alzheimer's.

However, just like at the gym, one single exercise is not going to exercise your whole brain. In the gym you do bicep curls for your biceps, push-ups for your chest and other exercises specific to particular muscle groups. Same goes for brain exercises. This is why I will list a variety of brain-related puzzles and exercises which will not only preserve what you have, but build on it. This is not hyperbole – *you really can make yourself smarter!*

Before we proceed, I need to reiterate the point I made earlier in the book – you need to ensure that you are giving any mental puzzles your full attention. Absentmindedly doing a puzzle while watching TV is not doing to do you much good. Give each puzzle your full attention and you will benefit accordingly.

## Ping pong
Yes, you read that correctly – ping pong!

This is probably the best sport you can play for your brain as it uses several important parts at the same time. The requirement for hand-eye co-ordination keeps your brain firing at top capacity. Part of your brain's functioning is related to speed, which ping pong helps grow as it pushes your brain to react quickly.

The second interesting aspect of ping pong is that it heavily relies on the basal ganglia, a part of your brain not only involved in movement but also in mood disorders. So a basal ganglia working in good order not only helps you maintain and improve hand-eye co-ordination, but keeps your mood up.

The final important aspect of ping pong is that it is not physically taxing on your joints unless you suffer from poor mobility already. There is little impact on your knees and ankles which should keep the probability of injuring yourself low.

## Mensa IQ puzzles

All my life I have enjoyed Mensa puzzles as a way to keep my brain running well. For those of you unfamiliar, Mensa is an organisation for people with high IQs. I always found it a bit too much like a 'status symbol' for smart people to feel better than others so never really got into the other aspects of Mensa. However their books with various puzzles and tests are second to none.

I always had to go out and buy Mensa puzzle books however now you have many more options which are often free. You can visit the Mensa web site (see the Resources section) or grab one of the Mensa apps from ITunes or the Google app store.

The beauty of these kinds of tests and puzzles is that they tax so many different parts of your brain at the same time. I really can't think of a better way to exercise your brain in such a comprehensive fashion than by doing puzzles and tests like these.

Don't forget, if you don't want to visit Mensa, just type "IQ Test" into your search engine to find many free options online.

I am not much of a believer in a static IQ that each person is born with that determines their success in life. I know of a lot of high IQ types who have generally struggled with leading a happy life and I know plenty of below-average IQ people who are great successes. That being said, it is immensely satisfying to do your first IQ test, keep practicing and then slowly building your IQ up. Naturally, part of this is because you are just getting better at IQ tests because you are familiar with them and can pick up patterns in the questions. However there is also a strong component that represents the fact that you *are* getting smarter, which is a great feeling.

## Sudoku, crosswords etc

These types of games are also very good for your brain. They are probably not as good as IQ tests in that they don't use as many different parts of your brain, however they still have an important place in your healthy brain lifestyle. The reason is that they are fun! The more enjoyable something is, the more likely you are to integrate it into your lifestyle. People can become absolute Sudoku fanatics!

## Chess and other 'strategic' board-games

Strategic games harness unique parts of your brain that other puzzles do not. Inherent in these games is the skill of thinking laterally and creatively. You not only need to predict your opponent's reaction to your move, but your subsequent reaction and then your opponent's subsequent reaction to that! Chess can be extremely mentally taxing – which is exactly what you want! Don't worry if you are no 'grand-master' – that is not the point. Try to find an opponent who is either around your level or a little better than you.

It doesn't matter what type of game you chose, it doesn't have to be chess. However the most important point is that you win by your own effort. Avoid any games with a strong 'luck' component as these will be counter-productive.

## Writing

The act of writing is extremely beneficial for your brain. Interestingly, fiction and nonfiction appear to have a small difference in how they benefit your brain. Fiction is good for fostering a strong imagination. You need to create everything from nothing, which is great for your brain. Nonfiction is also good for your brain as you need to draw information from memory and convey it in a clear and interesting way (something I hopefully have achieved – if not, sorry).

Writing a book is also good for your mood, as per the theory of *effort based rewards*. There is a tremendous sense of satisfaction which comes with completely a project such as a book. This is great for your mood.

## Reading nonfiction

If you are traditionally the type of person who either reads trashy romance or by-the-numbers thrillers or who doesn't read at all, expanding your mind with some nonfiction will be great for your brain. Try to pick something that you are interested in and is reasonably challenging. For example, in high school I had no interest in physics, however in recent times I have been fascinated by the subject so I have been burying myself in books on subatomic particles and quantum theory. Sometimes I have to re-read sentences multiple times to understand the topic! It is not only interesting to understand the fundamental laws of the universe, but I know I am doing my brain a favour at the same time.

# Conclusion

No single part of this book is going to suddenly give you a perfect brain. *Nothing* is going to suddenly give you a perfect brain. It takes time and effort and will require nothing short of your utmost patience. However, what I have hoped to achieve is –

- You now have a greater understanding of what is healthy and what is unhealthy for your brain

- This means that you can avoid unhealthy thinking and behaviours which were taking you backwards

- You can then engage in behaviours which will take you *forwards* instead

As I have mentioned several times, the key is attention and mindfulness. Without these qualities, you will not be able to derive full benefit from the activities and behaviours in this book. Attention will also ensure that you do not unconsciously drift back into bad habits without noticing.

If you follow all the recommendations in this book, in all but the most severe and refractory cases, I am confident that you will soon find yourself with a happier and healthier brain.

I wish you all the best.


Ps – If you think that others would benefit from this book, please consider leaving a review on Amazon here.

Also, if you enjoyed this book, please check out my other books and guides here on Amazon.

## Appendix 1 – Meditation Instructions

Here are some basic meditation instructions. I will concentrate on 'breath' meditation as it is well-suited to reducing physiological arousal associated with insomnia -

1.  Sit up in a comfortable position

2.  Take a few deep, slow breaths and concentrate on the sensation of air passing through your nostrils

3.  Count "one" on the 'in-breath' and "two" on the 'out-breath' all the way to "10" and then start again at "one".

4.  When you find your thoughts wandering, just start again at "one". A useful way to notice that your mind has wandered is when you say "eleven" – that's your sign to tell you that you have passed "ten" because you were thinking about something else.

5.  When your mind wanders (and it WILL wander), just bring it back to "one" and don't get frustrated. This is the number one mistake that beginners make. They think that the purpose of meditation is to completely stop thinking. This is impossible and is not the goal of meditation. The act of realising your mind has wandered and bringing it back to your breath - that is meditation.

6.  If you do this prior to bed, after a little while you will struggle to stay awake, so just lay down and enjoy the relaxed feeling. You will soon drop off to sleep.

# Resources

*Beyond Blue* – Australian government depression and anxiety resource page - www.beyondblue.org.au

*Crazy Meds* – interesting site and forum with down to earth, no bull information on various meds - www.crazymeds.us

*Alan Wallace homepage* – fantastic part Buddhism/part science site - http://www.alanwallace.org/

*Authentic Happiness* – site for ground-breaking psychologist Martin Seligman - http://www.authentichappiness.sas.upenn.edu/Default.aspx

*John Ratey* – Author of "Spark" – fantastic book on the effects of exercise on the brain – http://www.johnratey.com/newsite/index.html

*Daniel Goleman* – Author of "Emotional Intelligence" - http://www.danielgoleman.info/blog/

*Rick Hanson* – Author of "The Buddha's Brain" http://www.rickhanson.net/

*Thich Nhat Hanh* – legendary Vietnamese Zen Monk http://www.plumvillage.org/

*Ram Dass* – legendary spiritual teacher http://www.ramdass.org/

*Mensa Brain Test* - http://www.mensabraintest.com/index.html

www.ingramcontent.com/pod-product-compliance
Lightning Source LLC
Chambersburg PA
CBHW071724170526
45165CB00005B/2140